BODY PSYCHOTHERAPY

An Introduction

BODY PSYCHOTHERAPY

An Introduction

Nick Totton

Open University Press
Maidenhead · Philadelphia

Open University Press
McGraw-Hill Education
McGraw-Hill House
Shoppenhangers Road
Maidenhead
Berkshire
England
SL6 2QL

email: enquiries@openup.co.uk
world wide web: www.openup.co.uk

and
325 Chestnut Street
Philadelphia, PA 19106, USA

First Published 2003

A catalogue record of this book is available from the British Library

ISBN   0 335 21038 4 (pb)   0 335 21039 2 (hb)

Library of Congress Cataloging-in-Publication Data
Totton, Nick.
  Body psychotherapy: an introduction / Nick Totton.
    p. cm.
  Includes bibliographical references and index.
  ISBN 0-335-21039-2 – ISBN 0-335-21038-4 (pbk.)
  1. Mind and body therapies. 2. Psychotherapy. 3. Reich, Wilhelm,
  1897–1957. I. Title.
  RC489.M53 T68 2003
  616.89′14–dc21   2002035539

Typeset by Graphicraft Limited, Hong Kong
Printed and bound by CPI Group (UK) Ltd, Croydon, CR0 4YY

Contents

Foreword

How strange, how synchronistic, that at the precise moment Nick Totton asked me to write this foreword to what is certain to become the standard work on body psychotherapy, I slipped a disk between C5 and C6 in my upper spine. The MRI scan showed the protrusion clearly and the pain was as bad as anything I've experienced, with acute sensations referred down my entire right arm, wrist and hand.

As a psychotherapist, I am more or less programmed to look as deeply as I can into the likely causes and significance of this injury beyond, though definitely including, the physical and material dimension. I could see how my father's death a few months earlier, and some family unpleasantness surrounding it, might have been a factor. And the intense desire to take a prolonged break from all work, in particular from writing (I am right-handed), was also something to think about. Having recently got married, which also brings its inevitable challenges and responsibilities, I wanted to spend time with my wife and get off the wheel of intense commitment to studying and writing, engaging in politics and seeing clients to which I had become accustomed.

Having had body psychotherapy myself, I could also see how the symptoms perfectly expressed emotional states with which I am becoming increasingly familiar: the problems of ageing, a sense of having shouldered too great a burden, a desire to stop communicating indirectly by writing and to start to do it more directly via speech and touch, and a recognition that all the insights that come from a reasonably productive analysis can't prevent some kind of eruption when a parent dies in less than ideal circumstances.

Now the reason I am beginning this foreword in such a way is not to indulge mindlessly in self-disclosure or self-revelation or play some kind of charismatic game – 'look at me suffering but going on with my work', etc., etc. No, the reason is to show that, as an analytical psychotherapist (actually, a Jungian analyst), I am already completely within the realm of body psychotherapy whether I like it or not, whether I acknowledge it or not and whether I know anything about it or not (for I have not had one single dedicated hour of seminar study devoted specifically to it). In this sense, I am not atypical. Many 'verbal psychotherapists' know, or think they know, quite a bit about the body and its vicissitudes, and especially about the necessity to go beyond body-mind and body-spirit splits so as to embrace a more comprehensive vision of the human subject (if not always a holistic one when the cosmic and political backdrops to subject- ivity are overlooked, as they often are). In the twenty-first century, I simply could not have an identity as a psychotherapist, or feel remotely competent as such, without being able to traverse the fields of expres- sion and understanding I am clumsily referring to here.

So, given its covert ubiquity, what has happened both to *marginalize* body psychotherapy, and to bring it, as Nick Totton quite rightly puts it, to the threshold of a new paradigm and a new standing within the psychological healing arts?

As far as the demeanment of body psychotherapy goes, this can be attributed – as can so many distasteful and even grotesque practices and scenarios within the history of psychotherapy – to the seemingly unstoppable political project of orthodox (i.e. institutional) psychoana- lysis in its various but heavily interlinked guises. Wilhelm Reich became an embarrassment and, as important, a threat to Freudian leadership. (Much the same story can be seen in relation to Ferenczi and Jung though with different footnotes.) Reich's politics threatened to ruin the chances for acceptance on the part of psychoanalysis, which has always had an ambivalent relationship with power and the powerful. Moreover, Western societies are not at home with the body and this alienation increases the more sophisticated (and hence body-distant) modern medi- cine becomes with its battery of scans, systems, drugs and prostheses. A good proportion of body psychotherapy has been experienced as making a claim for a healing potential located within the body itself, one that comes on stream when facilitated to do so. This claim, which, if you think about it, decentres the therapist, explains why body psychotherapy found a home in the humanistic and human potential traditions of psychotherapy and is very threatening to comfortable habits of mind. The psychotherapy establishment has dealt with the claim by depicting the body psychotherapist variously as a potential abuser, left-wing fanatic, guru, or untrained enthusiast depending on who is doing the accusing. Nick Totton goes over all this ground in a scholarly way, including a pro- found discussion of the over-reaction on the part of body psychotherapists in terms of a search for spurious respectability, but it might help readers to have the position spelled out in these intemperate terms.

To return to the question of why body psychotherapy is at a threshold, I would like to offer some heuristic images concerning this. It is as if body psychotherapy has been either dozing or drugged or running on less than its full complement of cylinders, waiting for the discoveries that are being made by today's explorers in the fields of neuropsychoanalysis, neurobiology and brain research generally. As Nick Totton points out, the brain is part of the body and yet I have so far failed to find a single reference in the copious and growing literature that suggests that body-based psychotherapy might have anything to offer to support the much touted claim that psychotherapy, going over the ground of very early experiences, can actually influence brain structure and pattern for the good of the individual concerned, just as the parents' handling in infancy exerts such an influence.

In the remainder of this foreword, I'd like to focus on some themes in the book that seem to me to be particularly suggestive in that they show how contemporary body psychotherapy chimes with what is happening at the cutting edge of psychotherapy generally: the decline of 'insight' as the greatest good in psychotherapy; the impact of the cultural and political dimensions of experience on the psyche; spirituality and psychotherapy; and some thoughts about touch, contact and relationship.

There is a sense in which the popular image of the main gain of psychotherapy as being 'insight' will have to change. 'It's all to do with your mother' or 'you are constantly sabotaging your own conscious desires because of a sense of guilt' are not only, by now, bound to be the case, it just isn't where best practice in psychotherapy is headed. Whatever one calls it, the process of *exploration of what is the case*, rather than its interpretation, has moved more and more to the centre of psychotherapeutic endeavour. While it would be too simplistic to posit 'finding out what one feels' as the true function of psychotherapy, there is a growing recognition that it is to changes in what is experienced and how it is experienced (and expressed, whether by word or bodily motion) that we must look to find out what is interesting in the therapy project. Meaning turns out to involve something other than 'meaning'. The body is an absolutely perfect arena for this kind of 'phenomenological' exploration. Some call it 'here and now', others 'the present unconscious'; I prefer to speak of 'things as they seem to be'.

Another huge shift in the psychotherapy world is the recognition that culture, and, in particular, political arrangements of all kinds impact on what used to be regarded as 'private' in significant ways. Nick Totton's previous outstanding work on psychotherapy and politics has clearly prepared him to develop such ideas, both in terms of recognizing these fields as factors in therapy and as a communicator and even advocate of the perspective. The body is so utterly caught up in what is by no means 'natural' that therapy with body in mind turns out to be extremely politically and culturally sensitive. In fact, with the rising interest in transcultural and intercultural psychotherapy, it is only a matter of time before the immense cultural differences in attitude to body come to be seen as a positive advantage rather than a disadvantage for the psychotherapist committed to working with and through the body. All bodies are different from one perspective or another and so the cultural difference angle is also of relevance to psychotherapy situations where differences are not necessarily obvious.

The body is not only a site where we will find compliance with culture and its dictates, meaning the majority culture and, in Western countries, the market-driven, consumerist, conformist version of culture. The body is also in protest against such trends, even, or so it can be argued, a prime site of resistance to the homogenizing and globalizing facets of contemporary life. Sometimes this protest will lead to states of discomfort and even disease but, at least as I understand it, a good-enough body psychotherapist will be careful before pathologizing somatic symptoms prematurely without understanding their radical and resistant nature (which links us back to my disk problem, not to mention the array of so-called 'psychosomatic disorders', appetite disorders, addictions, and so on).

Much contemporary psychotherapy, including splinter elements of psychoanalysis but mainly in the integrative and humanist traditions, is engaging with the spiritual dimension of life, sometimes under the banner of 'transpersonal psychotherapy'. Nick Totton states that 'the more deeply one goes into the experience of embodiment, the more strongly one becomes aware of the spiritual and subtle aspects of reality'. I agree with this (and in another place I put forward the idea of a 'profane spirituality', basing it on Richard Zaehner's notion of profane mysticism). Totton suggests that it is in the importance that body psychotherapy often gives to breathing that one finds the most palpable link to spirit – breath, *pneuma*, *ruach*, spirit. Another link that interests me is in the idea of 'surrender', whether to body processes or to the numinous/divine/awesome/wholly other. I think that the idea of surrender is different from some sort of masochistic self-abnegation or submission. These might well be considered, as the Jungian analyst Rosemary Gordon once put it, as the shadow side of the desire to worship and feel reverent. The relational psychoanalyst Emmanuel Ghent has argued that there could be a dialogical element in spiritual experience even when the human subject is confronted with the 'bigger' entities. Jung, too, in his work on Job, makes it clear that in such a dialogue, God will benefit because human consciousness possesses some things (mainly to do with suffering and its gifts) that even He does not.

The final theme that I would like to single out concerns the links between 'touch', 'contact' and 'relationship'. As a Jungian analyst, I have been encouraged to take the view that physical touch is not a *sine qua non* for contact and relationship. And I do still believe in that, though I can see that it is a somewhat abstract and idealized position. For increasingly, I find that if there is no bodily aspect at all in a therapy relationship, the relationship has to fight harder to really deliver the goods for the persons within it. I am not sure if physical touch is the only bodily dimension that can add something to psychotherapy – I have had some experience with utilizing spontaneous movement within an analytical frame that has made me see that it is *body itself* rather than touch that is the important factor. Be that as it may, I think that it is the connection of body to relationship within a world starved of, and looking for, authentic relating (whether on the personal or collective levels) that should engage our attention as psychotherapists and as human beings.

Andrew Samuels

Introduction

Behind your thoughts and feelings, my brother, there stands a mighty ruler, an unknown sage – whose name is self. In your body he dwells; he is your body.

(Nietzsche 1978: 34)

Body psychotherapy is an idea whose time has come – again. When I started practising in Leeds in the 1970s, there were four Reichian therapists living within an area of three streets – a situation which may be unique in world history; our clients assumed that there were body therapists everywhere. Since that point, body psychotherapy has fallen drastically out of fashion; but recently it has begun to attract new interest, for reasons which are no doubt complex, but which probably include the steadily increasing formalization and schematization of psychotherapy trainings. Students are starting to feel that there is something missing. They are seeking out body psychotherapy workshops and courses, and asking for such work to be included in their training.

This book is partly for those students, and for psychotherapy practitioners who similarly want to expand their range of knowledge; but also for clients and potential clients – for anyone who feels that their bodily experience is less satisfying and pleasurable than it should be, or that their body is trying to tell them something in a language they do not quite understand. This book exists to let them know that they are right; and that there is something they can do about it.

I am also writing for body psychotherapists themselves, who often do not have a sufficiently rich and subtle conceptual understanding of what they do intuitively; or who, like other psychotherapy practitioners, may have large gaps in their knowledge beyond the specific school in which they were trained. I have tried to produce a picture of the whole field, and of how each specific form of work is situated within it. I have also tried to provide a wider context of other initiatives in our culture towards a revaluation of embodiment – a context which turns out to support the traditional beliefs of body psychotherapy in an almost uncanny way.

One reader of a draft version of this book commented several times 'your politics are showing'. I make no apology for this; but I hope that it becomes apparent that it is not just my personal idiosyncratic politics (though no doubt there are elements of this) but a politics that follows naturally from the central understandings of body psychotherapy. And this, I would suggest, is the other reason why body psychotherapy is again of interest: because our situation needs it. We have reached a cultural point where the body itself is under threat, from many directions. Body psychotherapy is one rallying point for resistance to these threats.

It is only one of many such points, of course; and many people who learn body psychotherapy move on to something else, a situation which seems to me very healthy. My own trainer is now a lecturer in counselling. His own trainer is a midwife. (His trainer, in turn, was Ola Raknes, who was trained by Wilhelm Reich.) Many of my own trainees now work in a wide range of other fields. In these sorts of ways the experience of embodied relationship, and everything that goes with it, are spread through the culture as a transformative yeast.

I want to thank Roz Carroll, Em Edmondson, Hélène Fletcher, Keith Pearce and Courtenay Young, all of whom read and commented on draft sections of this book – and none of whom, of course, are responsible for what I have finally written. And I want to dedicate the book to my body psychotherapy community – all my clients, therapists, trainees, trainers, supervisors, supervisees and peers: with deep gratitude.

I have used 'she' and 'her' in what follows to represent the generic human. Several quoted passages using 'he' and 'him' have been left unchallenged. I have tried to avoid referring to research which harms animals.

CHAPTER I

What happens in body psychotherapy?

As feelings rush up during the session or exercise, a deep rhythm from the system tries to impose itself and, since the rhythm is more fluent, more coherent than the personality, it will run into blocks posing as attitudes.

(Grossinger 1995, Vol. 2: 194)

This chapter is intended particularly for readers with little or no personal experience of body psychotherapy, whether as clients or as practitioners. Hopefully it will also be of interest to those more familiar with the field. In it, I try so far as is possible to convey the flavour of the work, beginning with some body psychotherapy sessions which are, I think, representative – despite (or possibly because of) being fictional. Case histories and vignettes are of course always in a sense fictional. So much needs changing for reasons of confidentiality, or simplifying for reasons of comprehensibility, that they can never fully describe the reality of what takes place. It seemed simpler therefore to construct some useful fictions to illustrate the range of body psychotherapy work. The chapter moves on to look at accounts of body psychotherapy by clients and by practitioners themselves and finishes with a discussion of the sorts of goals and outcomes which all of these imply.

In this chapter in particular, I want to encourage readers to bear in mind that reading about therapy is always stirring; and reading about body psychotherapy, particularly if you have never experienced it, is particularly so. You will be reacting in part mentally, but also in an *embodied* way, with feelings, sensations and impulses to movement. All of this is valuable information, which can enormously enrich your understanding of what you are reading. So go slowly, breathe, and let yourself have your reactions.

Six sessions

The following descriptions of therapy sessions are all imaginary, and not based on any specific clients (or practitioners). Each, though, is fairly typical of a particular style of body psychotherapy. They are intended to give a simplified impression of some of the sorts of things that are likely to happen when people do body psychotherapy together.

Session one

Alan arrives for his weekly session with his therapist, Judith, with what he describes as a 'blinding headache'. He starts to tell her about his week, but the headache makes it hard for him to concentrate. 'Perhaps we should focus on this headache first?' Judith suggests. 'Can you tell me more about exactly what it feels like?'

Alan is familiar from previous sessions with focusing on bodily states. He pauses to clarify his internal perception of his headache, and Judith notices that as he does so he screws up his eyes and pulls his head and neck back into his shoulders, tortoise-fashion. 'I feel it mostly around my eyes and forehead,' he explains slowly. 'It's a stabbing pain . . . As if someone was driving a nail into my forehead.'

'Perhaps you could show me?' Judith suggests. 'Show me how you would do that to me – how you would drive a nail in to make me feel that sort of pain.' She stands up and Alan responds by standing up and moving over to her. He mimes holding a nail to her forehead between her eyes and hammering it in with his other hand. With each 'hammer blow' he makes a growling sound, pulling his teeth back as he does so.

Judith briefly considers a few alternatives. She could ask Alan to make more noise, and support him in a stronger physical expression of aggressiveness and violence; it might be that suppressed anger is behind his headache. She could also explore with him whether there is a relationship issue involved here: Alan seems very involved in 'hurting' her, and perhaps this is expressing something important about the therapeutic situation. What she decides to do, though (and this decision only takes a few seconds) is to explore directly the 'purpose' of the headache.

'So I'm Alan, and you're now Alan's headache – you're the part of yourself who's giving him the headache,' she suggests. 'Can you tell him why you need him to have this headache?' She speaks directly as 'Alan' to the 'headache-maker': 'Why are you doing this to me? What do you need?'

Alan lets himself respond instinctively, without working it out. 'I'm trying to distract you,' he growls. 'I need you to stop thinking about things. Stop it now! STOP THINKING!' As he gets more and more impassioned, he carries on 'hammering' at Judith's forehead.

'What will happen if I think?' Judith asks, still in the role of 'Alan'. 'What is it I mustn't think about?'

'About Sue!' Alan shouts. Sue is his partner. 'Stop thinking about—'

'About what?'

'About leaving Sue!' Alan is shocked by what he has said. He stops 'hammering' and stands, breathing deeply and looking a bit dazed. Judith suggests that they both sit down again, and stays quiet, giving him time to recover. She remembers that when he arrived Alan described his headache as 'blinding'. Now they both know what it was meant to blind him *to*, she thinks. Although on the one hand he wants to end his long-term relationship with Sue, he is also frightened about the consequences and would rather not 'see' his own dissatisfaction.

As they start to talk this through, Judith feels dissatisfied. She starts to feel a slight headache herself. Experience tells her that this sort of symptom – especially when it echoes the client's process in this way – is generally there to alert her to something. What is it, she asks herself? Then she realizes 'in a blinding flash' that she and Alan have both been treating his headache as essentially negative, a force which is trying to cover up his real feelings. This is not how Judith thinks of symptoms in general. In her experience, they always have a positive, creative function if understood fully. And, she further realizes, in this case the positive function of the headache was to bring Alan's 'blindness' to the attention of both of them: to open things up to the light, rather than to hide them away.

When she shares this new viewpoint with Alan, though, it creates some tension. He resents what he sees as her tendency to 'think too much' about every detail of what happens. 'Well,' Judith points out, 'that's what you were saying when you were hammering away at my head – "Stop thinking!" Perhaps it really was *my* head you were hammering at, as well as "Alan's"?' Yet another aspect of Alan's symptom emerges: its relevance to issues in the therapeutic relationship, which will be taken up in further sessions.

Session two

Clare arrives on time for her session with Marsha and follows the usual pattern which has developed between them: after a few minutes to say hallo, re-establish their relationship and share any important news, Clare moves from her chair to the mattress and lies on her back. Marsha kneels quietly beside her, and Clare relaxes, brings her attention within herself, and starts to focus on her breathing. Early in their work together, she felt very strange and self-conscious at this point, but by now it feels reassuring and safe, an important part of her week.

'Yes,' Marsha says softly, as she has often said before, 'just relax, let your breathing happen – invite it to deepen a little, go just a little further with each outbreath, each inbreath.'

Clare finds her breath responding to Marsha's encouragement without any conscious effort on her part. As her breathing deepens, she feels her body 'wake up' in response to the extra energy running through it. Her arms and legs start to tingle slightly, and she becomes warmer. 'My throat feels tight,' Clare says. She coughs once or twice, and rubs her throat with her hand.

'How about if I do that for you?' Marsha suggests. When Clare nods, she puts her own hand gently on Clare's throat and rubs upwards towards her jaw. Marsha is feeling sensitively for the tension in her client's throat, and soon a bout of deeper coughing is provoked, with Clare's body jackknifing slightly at the waist. 'Yes, that's it, let it come,' Marsha encourages, knowing that – unlike some people – Clare responds positively to verbal support. 'Let the sound come through.' Clare's cough turns into something more like a growling roar, but to Marsha it sounds muffled and she notices that Clare is squeezing her hands into fists and raising her shoulders. Marsha quickly finds a small cushion to give her, and Clare squeezes and twists the cushion as she yells and shouts more freely. Using her hands like this helps to open up her voice, as if she is moving the 'strangling' impulse down from her own throat into her hands and out into the cushion.

'Are there any words in there?' Marsha asks. She suspects that it is not just angry sound in general which Clare has 'strangled', but specific angry statements. At first there is no response, but when she asks again, Clare starts to repeat, 'Leave me alone, leave me ALONE,' squeezing the cushion in rhythm with her words. After a while the volume starts to ease off, and Clare gradually relaxes until she is lying back weeping gently and still whispering 'Leave me alone.' Marsha murmurs encouragement and support, and strokes her arm. After another minute, Clare takes a deep, spontaneous breath and relaxes fully. Her breathing is even, full and calm. Her eyes are closed. Marsha waits patiently until Clare is ready of her own accord to 'come back into the room' and talk about what has happened, making connections with issues and themes in her life.

Session three

James has been in twice-weekly therapy for two years, focusing especially on his father's physical violence towards him when he was small, and the ways in which this has affected James's life. Alan, his therapist, knows that there is a lot of pain stored in James's body, but he has been very cautious about tapping into it, since he does not want to restimulate James's feelings until the situation feels safe enough to contain them. However, the two of them have recently worked through a lot of James's suspicion and mistrust of Alan, so Alan has been wondering whether some of James's traumatic material might be going to make itself felt. Partway through the session James says, 'I'm feeling quite frightened. Not of you, though – I trust you a lot more now. But there's a nagging fear in the background, under the surface.'

'How do you know that you're frightened?' Alan asks. 'I mean, what are you experiencing that feels like fear?' He is inviting James to connect with his bodily experience and this is what happens.

'Well, I'm feeling cold,' James replies slowly, 'and I have butterflies in my tummy, except they feel more sinister than butterflies . . . Can't catch my breath properly . . . Chest feels strange . . .'

'Strange how?'

'Like . . . Like . . . It feels frozen. Black. Feels like a frozen black lake . . .' James is becoming distressed.

Alan can see that he is pale, breaking into a sweat and his voice is laboured as if he is struggling to breathe. Alan keeps his response calm and relaxed. 'Uh-huh. That's great, James. A frozen black lake. Just stay relaxed and tell me, what would be the *opposite* of that image? Can you visualize something that is the opposite of a frozen black lake? What comes to mind?'

James is silent for a moment. 'A sunrise . . . What I see is a sunrise – you know, all red and orange and yellow, everything opening up and warming up . . .'

'Good, a sunrise, that's beautiful. Stay with that image, James. And tell me what you're experiencing in your body now,' Alan says.

'Still cold, but it feels a little easier.' James is visibly less distressed, but still pale and constricted. His breath has become deeper. 'Not butterflies in my tummy . . . Bats . . . Like bats in the belfry! Trying to fly up into my chest . . .'

'Is it OK to let them fly up? Fly up into the sunrise?'

James pauses to check this out internally. 'Yes, it feels OK . . . I'm letting them fly up . . . Makes everything shaky though . . .'

Alan can see that James's chest and torso are indeed starting to tremble. He recognizes this as a positive sign that the body is discharging stored distress. 'Great, James, that's fine – let the shaking happen . . . Let the bats fly up and away . . . Let yourself shake, yes, that's great, let it spread.' The tremour spreads from James's chest into his shoulders and arms, becoming stronger and fuller. Alan supports and encourages James in allowing this, until it dies away naturally. James is breathing in deep sighs which gradually settle down along with the shaking. His eyes have closed.

'How are you feeling, James?'

'Good,' James says slowly. 'I feel pretty good . . . Strange but good. Relaxed.' Alan knows that they have embarked on the next stage of their journey together. Eventually James may connect up his bodily sensations and his imagery with memories of painful events, but this can come gradually, in its own time.

Session four

Carole is a psychotherapist with a background in dance and movement. Alison, here for her third weekly session, is starting to talk about how much she dislikes her body. 'It's too big, too fat, too heavy. I hate how clumsy and awkward it is – I hate how it lumbers about, knocking into people.'

Carole notices that Alison is moving around a lot on the sofa as she says this, acting out what she describes; and also that, although there is clearly real upset here, there is also something humorous and parodic about it. 'Why don't you show me what it's like?' Carole suggests. 'This big, clumsy, awkward body – how does it move?'

Carole stands up herself, as encouragement, and Alison quite willingly follows her lead. She starts to act out what she is describing, heaving herself around the room in a caricature performance. Carole – herself a large woman – joins in, mirroring back Alison's movements in a way which amplifies them, and soon the two women are cavorting around the room together, laughing wildly. 'The Dance of the Fatties!' Alison calls out. She is clearly having fun, but there is also something very serious about it and Carole starts to perceive something quite aggressive and animal-like in the movements Alison is producing.

As Carole mirrors this new quality, Alison picks it up in her own movement. Carole draws back and gives Alison the space – 'You carry on, show me the feeling' – and something like a gorilla starts to emerge. Alison begins to beat her chest and to make a snarling face. 'Is there a sound with this?' Carole asks, and Alison growls and roars at her for a few minutes. Carole joins in again, so there are two gorillas posturing and growling at each other. Again the dance becomes funny and after a minute both women are laughing and exhausted and it feels natural to sit down.

'So the Dance of the Fatties is also the Dance of the Gorillas?' Carole comments. 'It seems as though this body that lumbers around and knocks into people might be quite aggressive. What do you think it's angry about?'

'While I was roaring and beating my chest,' Alison says, 'I was thinking: Don't mess with me! If you mess with me I'll smash you to pieces!'

'Is that how you generally relate to people?' Carole asks. She is fairly sure of the answer, but doesn't yet know Alison very well.

'No, not at all. My friends tell me I let people walk all over me.'

'I wonder – if you looked after yourself better, perhaps you might start to experience your body a bit differently,' Carole suggests. 'You said that you hate the way it lumbers about knocking into people; but maybe it's just saying "I deserve to take up space"? Walking over other people instead of being walked over . . .'

Alison is plainly unenthusiastic about this way of understanding her attitude to herself; and Carole is well aware that she is speculating – she doesn't yet know Alison well enough to be confident that she has got it right. But it's clear that they have found a way of exploring together which is useful and creative for both of them.

Session five

Chloe arrives a little late and her therapist, Andrew, experiences her as absent and confused. She tells a rambling story about driving through heavy traffic, then trails off.

'Are you OK?' Andrew asks. 'You seem a bit preoccupied.'

'I do feel strange,' Chloe agrees, rubbing her head. 'I feel as though something important is about to happen, but I don't know what it is. It feels ominous – something big I've got to go through . . . But I don't know what's on the other side.'

As they talk, it gradually dawns on Andrew that Chloe's state is familiar from work with other clients. She describes a feeling of pressure in her head and continues to talk about an ominous sense of having to 'go through something'. Both of these elements, in Andrew's experience, point towards some sort of 'birth process' being underway, as he would put it to himself – some sort of reliving of Chloe's experience of being born. Meanwhile, Chloe is becoming somewhat distressed, flushed and incoherent.

'Can we try something?' he suggests. 'Lie down here, on your side, and if it's OK with you I'm going to hold your head like this. Let me know if you want me to stop.' He cups the top of Chloe's head in his hands and applies a gentle, rhythmic compression. His suspicion is confirmed when Chloe's head immediately and spontaneously pushes back against his hands, and her breathing changes.

'Yes!' Chloe says strongly. 'That feels right . . . That's what my body needs to do.' By trial and error, they settle into a position with Andrew kneeling at Chloe's head, while her feet are firmly anchored against the side of the sofa. Encouraged by Andrew, Chloe pushes harder and harder against his hands, and he has to put his back into resisting her as she huffs and grunts more and more loudly, her body contracting and arching as she forces her way between his legs. Andrew resists enough to make it hard work for Chloe to get through, but yields to her tremendous effort, coming up onto his knees to make a sufficient space.

After 20 minutes, Chloe has successfully been 'born'. Eyes closed, and with an expression of unearthly peace on her face, she is cradled in Andrew's lap, breathing gently and calmly – while Andrew hopes that she can come round soon enough to make way for his next client . . .

Session six

We have already encountered Clare and her therapist Marsha in Session two. A few weeks later, after their usual initial talk Clare lies down on the mattress, and Marsha is about to kneel beside her to begin the body-work session. As she does so, though, Marsha's attention is caught by something different about her client. She experiences Clare's posture as stiff and reluctant and picks up a hint of fear in her eyes, as if the look of a hunted animal is hiding within Clare's gaze.

'Are you sure you want to do this?' Marsha asks. 'Maybe we should think about whether bodywork is the right way to go this week.' At first Clare does not admit to any reluctance and Marsha starts to wonder whether she is imagining it. When she considers returning to their usual structure, it feels as though it would be false and without real contact between them. As she is accustomed to doing, she brings her awareness to her own bodily state, and realizes that she feels tense and slightly sick. She cannot override her intuition that Clare is deeply unwilling. 'Just indulge me,' Marsha suggests. 'Take the time to feel what you're feeling. Take a good look at me and notice what you see.'

Clare follows Marsha's suggestion and realizes that she is indeed feeling quite strange and uncomfortable – the familiar routine of the session had obscured this from her. As she deepens into her own experience she starts to tremble, and Marsha's eyes become huge, dark and alien. Clare's head turns involuntarily from side to side in a 'NO' headshake gesture and she starts to pant. 'It's OK,' Marsha says gently. 'I'm not going to hurt you. Do you want to tell me what's happening?'

'I don't really know,' Clare mutters. 'Can't make sense of it . . . You look strange . . . Alien . . . Like a UFO being.'

'What do you want to say to me?'

'Stay away from me . . . Stay AWAY! Leave me ALONE!' With increasing intensity, Clare shouts at Marsha as she moves into a tight ball, as far away as she can get on the mattress, hands over her head. Marsha realizes that Clare seems to be revisiting the same material as in the previous session, where she was also saying 'Leave me alone'; but while previously she was expressing anger and grief, this time fear is the dominant emotion.

Also – and very importantly – while in the previous session Clare was treating Marsha as an ally in her imaginary encounter with important people from her past, now she is experiencing Marsha herself as the threatening 'alien'. This represents a valuable deepening of the work, but also means that the therapeutic relationship is more delicate. Marsha's experience tells her that direct bodywork of the kind they have been using will probably need to take a back seat for a while now. It would be too open to misinterpretation by the very vulnerable part of Clare which has come to the surface. They will need to work verbally for a while, exploring issues of transference and projection so as to build a firm container for further bodywork in the future.

What was that about?

It should be clear from the above that while body psychotherapists do some things which verbal psychotherapists don't do – and naturally I have emphasized these – they also do everything which verbal psychotherapists do. There is nothing in verbal psychotherapy which is inappropriate or irrelevant to body-focused work. Like verbal therapists, body psychotherapists talk with their clients, explore their process, pay particular attention to the therapeutic relationship, and try to help clients make sense of their experience. Central concepts and techniques like unconditional regard, here-and-now focus, owning projections, or analysing the transference are all just as applicable to body psychotherapy as to verbally based work.

These sessions are also slightly idealized. Like verbal therapists, body psychotherapists have plenty of sessions where nothing much seems to be happening. Good body psychotherapists, like good therapists of any kind, do not push their clients into certain kinds of experience. Exactly because bodily process can be quite overwhelming, most body therapists are especially careful to let the client decide at every point what is right for them, and to control the pace and depth of what happens. Some of the sessions I have described would only take place after a considerable time has been spent building trust and safety between the two people involved.

In the course of this book, I will be offering a context for understanding what these sessions are about: the thinking behind them, the aim and meaning of the techniques being used, and what leads people to respond in the ways I have illustrated. I will be trying to suggest why body psychotherapy is often a good way of exploring and resolving our issues; what sorts of problems it can help with; and what sorts of people it suits. The answers to all of these questions stem from the fundamental belief underlying body psychotherapy: that what we call 'mind' and 'body' are best understood as just different aspects of the same thing.

The client's tale

These were fictional sessions, but is there information available about what real body psychotherapy sessions are like? As we shall see, there are many excellent accounts by practitioners. First, though, we will look at *clients'* own reports of their experience of body psychotherapy.

One of the fullest descriptions, and almost certainly the funniest, is by Orson Bean (a well-known American film actor who appears, for example, in *Being John Malkovich*). His book *Me And The Orgone* (Bean 1971) describes an experience of classic Reichian body therapy – orgonomy – with Elsworth Baker in New York in the 1960s. This is from his first session:

> 'Lie down on the bed,' said the doctor. 'Yes, sure,' said Willie the Robot, and did so. 'Just breathe naturally,' he said, pulling a chair over to the bed and sitting down next to me. I fixed my eyes on a spot of water damage near the upper left-hand corner of Doctor Baker's window and breathed naturally. I thought: 'What if I get an erection, or shit on his bed or vomit.' The doctor was feeling the muscles around my jaw and neck. He found a tight cord in my neck, pressed it hard and kept on pressing it. It hurt like hell but Little Lord Jesus, no crying he makes.
>   'Did that hurt?' asked Doctor Baker.
>   'Well, a little,' I said, not wanting to be any trouble.
>
> (Bean 1971: 18)

Later in the session, though, things improve:

> 'All right,' said Baker. 'Now I want you to continue breathing and do a bicycle kick on the bed with your legs.' I began to raise my legs and bring them down rhythmically, striking the bed with my calves. My thighs began to ache, and I wondered when he would say that I had done it long enough, but he didn't. On and on I went, until my legs were ready to drop off. Then, gradually, it didn't hurt any more and that same sweet fuzzy sensation of pleasure began to spread through my whole body, only much stronger. I now felt as if a rhythm had taken over my kicking which had nothing to do with any effort on my part. I felt transported and in the grip of something larger than myself. I was breathing more deeply than I ever had before and I felt the sensation of each breath all the way down past my lungs and into my pelvis. Gradually, I felt myself lifted out of Baker's milk chocolate room and up into the spheres. I was beating to an astral rhythm. Finally, I knew it was time to stop. I lay there for how many minutes I don't know and I heard his voice say, 'How do you feel?'
>   'Wonderful,' I said. 'Is this always what happens?'
>   'More or less,' he said. 'I can see you on Tuesdays at two.'
>
> (Bean 1971: 20)

This, of course, is the beginning rather than the end of the therapy, but many people (including myself) have had similarly blissful experiences.

As Marvin Spiegelman, a Jungian analyst who received Reichian therapy and wrote a book about it, says: 'I sometimes even had mystical experiences on that Reichian couch – profound feelings of oneness with the universe, the benevolence of God, the unity of life . . . Reichian work enhances this experience of cosmic energy, with or without specific content or imagery' (1992: 203).

Richard Grossinger's account of body psychotherapy is more poetic but essentially similar.

> As mind and body flow together, and achieve their nondifference, tension momentarily lightens . . . The blossoms on the trees hang as globes of fuzzy light, expanding eternally without weight and made of tenderness more than of matter. Memories that seemed to have been lost forever flood back in delicate sensings. Life becomes so large and expanded in their return that it is itself sufficient and ample; there is enough to drink forever, but there is not so much that one would drown. One's size changes, the sense of being cramped in a body softens. The torso expands to hold a figure which is a once more muscular and firm and more angelic and graceful. For the duration of the feeling, lost functions are intuited and sometimes even recovered.
>
> (Grossinger 1995, Vol. 2: 196–7)

Michael Eigen is a well-known American psychoanalyst who underwent body psychotherapy with Stanley Keleman – something which, he says, 'supplemented my personal analysis and opened ways of experiencing I otherwise might not have reached' (Eigen 1993: xviii). His description is couched in objective terms, but derives from personal experience:

> As one breathes more deeply into one's tensions, streams of erotic sensations may be triggered off . . . Feelings of power and energy rise and fall and become concentrated in particular body zones as well as remaining unpredictably fluid. The person first experiences a defensive consciousness in relation to the rise of body feelings. The ego is interested in, stimulated and frightened by the unanticipated world of continuous and varied body sensations and feelings it begins to glimpse. A testing process evolves in which the ego gradually builds courage to tolerate and experiment with larger doses of being 'in' it. It gradually becomes an explorer of the shifting centers and currents of body aliveness.
>
> (Eigen 1993: 44)

Later in this book we will be giving these personal narratives a theoretical and technical context in which to understand them. We also have available some more standardized information about clients' assessment of body psychotherapy. William West (1994) sent a questionnaire to 150 ex-clients of body psychotherapists who were members of Energy Stream (the Post Reichian Therapy Association), a small UK training organization. Of these clients 68 (45 per cent) returned a completed questionnaire – a limited sample, but sufficient to be of interest. The most important finding is that the proportion declaring themselves 'satisfied' or 'highly satisfied' with their experience of body psychotherapy was 77 per cent, closely in line with the general finding that around 80 per cent of psychotherapy clients are happy with their therapy. In other words, body psychotherapy seems to be as effective, from the client's perspective, as other forms of therapy, in the view of clients who have selected it as their preferred modality. No respondents described themselves as 'highly dissatisfied'; 9 per cent were 'dissatisfied' and the remainder neutral.

This finding conforms with the general tendency of research to show that all modalities of psychotherapy are roughly as effective as each other (Luborsky et al. 1985; Roth and Fonagy 1996: 341–57; Seligman 1995), and that the major factor which increases the effectiveness of therapy as perceived by both clients and professionals is the success of the therapeutic alliance – how helpful and sympathetic the therapist is experienced as being (Roth and Fonagy 1996: 350–5). In understanding these results, however, we need to remember that a majority of clients choose, at least to some degree, what form of therapy they undertake. Presumably those who knowingly come to a body psychotherapist, for example, already have a fairly strong sense that this approach will be helpful for them. Body psychotherapists are offering an unusual modality in an almost exclusively private setting, so many of their clients have actively sought them out.

Respondents were asked to rate the helpfulness of various therapeutic techniques, including several specific to bodywork. About two-thirds said that the use of breathing, massage or physical contact, and facilitating awareness of body energy were helpful or very helpful. This in fact represented the vast majority of those who reported these techniques being used – about a quarter of respondents had little or no experience of these methods. Like other 'body psychotherapists', these Energy Stream therapists were in fact holistic therapists who endeavour to use whatever techniques are appropriate for a particular client at a particular time – which does not always include direct bodywork.

Working with feelings is perhaps a feature in one way or another of almost all psychotherapies; but it is particularly central to body psycho-therapy, as we shall see in what follows, because of the role of emotion as a unique bridge between soma and psyche. Well over 90 per cent reported that the therapist had helped them both identify and express feelings. Nearly as many said that identifying feelings was helpful or very helpful, and 82.5 per cent said the same of expressing feelings. Interest-ingly, only 30 per cent felt that the therapist had helped them to *control* their feelings; and only two-thirds of these found it helpful. Possibly these figures would have been higher had they been asked about *management* rather than control of emotions. 'Exploring/accepting/expressing feelings' was identified as the particularly valuable feature of the therapy by 31 per cent of respondents, far higher than any other single element.

West also invited clients to offer metaphors for the therapeutic process (as I will discuss later, body psychotherapy often brings up very strong imagery). He groups these around the following main themes: 'elements (water, (sun)light, fire, earth); transformation, e.g. bud opening; animals; earth/concrete; journeys; womb/birth images'. He gives one eloquent example which incorporates several of these: 'In my first session I remember seeing myself as a black hole. Towards the end of my therapy I saw myself as a gold line. I see it as a journey from a dark claustrophobic watery hole, to the top of the water, and I splash out as a golden fish' (West 1994: 300).

The practitioner's tale

As I have already indicated, there are many excellent accounts of the practice of body psychotherapy written by practitioners. Some of the best of these are by Wilhelm Reich himself (for example, [1942] 1983: 309–29, which I have discussed in some detail in Totton 1999: 108–12; [1942] 1983: 350–4, discussed in Chapter 4; and Reich's extended description of therapy with a woman diagnosed as schizophrenic, [1950] 1972: 399–502). Some other recommended case studies and verbatim narratives can be found in Heckler (1984); Johnson (1997, especially the chapters by Conrad Da'oud and Hall); Johnson and Grand (1998); Levine (1997); Lowen (1976); Marrone (1990); and Mindell and Mindell (1992).

Here, though, rather than quoting briefly from a range of authors, I want to concentrate at some length on one particular case history out of all those available, in order to convey something of the flavour of how body practitioners approach their work – the issues and themes which arise, the questions they ask themselves, the goals they recognize. I have chosen an account by Emilie Conrad Da'oud (now Emilie Conrad), an American practitioner who as it happens (and as we shall see this reflects an important reality of the field) is not conventionally speaking a body *psychotherapist* as such. Conrad Da'oud is a dancer who has developed a form of body-centred practice which she calls Continuum.

In a chapter of *Groundworks: Narratives of Embodiment* (Johnson 1997), she describes her work with 'Barbara', a young woman who, when Conrad Da'oud met her, had been paraplegic since a car accident some years earlier. This is a situation which perhaps few body psychotherapists encounter, but despite this, and although of course every practitioner has their own style and predilections, I think that Conrad Da'oud's account gives a particularly vivid and meaningful picture of the reality of body psychotherapy, and in particular the complex relationship between the somatic and the psychological aspects of this work. She conveys the tremendous intimacy of body-focused practice, while maintaining a clear therapeutic perspective.

I can only quote extracts from Conrad Da'oud's account here since it covers a therapeutic relationship of some 20 years. When Conrad Da'oud first met Barbara, some 11 years after her injury, she says: 'I felt that after all these years she was still in great shock' (1997: 67). As we shall see, the concept of shock and the associated concept of trauma are of great importance in modern body psychotherapy. Conrad Da'oud argues that, under threat,

> we revert to an animal response by holding our breath in order to stop movement . . . In cases of severe trauma the threat does not seem to pass, and the protecting breath maintains its stasis. The shock is held in the breath and becomes patterned into the nervous system.
>
> (1997: 67)

For Conrad Da'oud, as for many other practitioners, working with the breath is the gateway to dissolving shock. Working with Barbara,

> I found her breath trapped high in her chest, much like a bird caught in a too tight cage, desperately flapping its wings to escape. I tracked how these new breaths began to interrupt the mad fluttering . . . The new breath creates an interference in the closed adaptation. This interference can now become a wedge that can continue to interrupt the stasis.
>
> (1997: 67)

With breath as a basis, Conrad Da'oud and her client began to explore what capacity for movement still remained in the system:

> Breath will stimulate intrinsic movement. Small undulating movements could be seen all through Barbara's torso and throat . . . She thought these subtle movements were interesting but of little consequence; after all, what do such twitches in the chest area have to do with walking? Like most people in wheelchairs, all Barbara's attention went to her legs. She was obsessed with walking, which was understandable, but her question was, how does one get from here to there? . . . I explained that movement begins intrinsically, and eventually, when strengthened, would become extrinsic, more dynamic and more functional. *In other words, walking begins with intrinsic movements of the spine, where the origin of 'legness' lies.*
>
> (1997: 67–8)

Conrad Da'oud describes how physical and energetic contact can facilitate this process:

> I held my hands over her spine, sometimes actually touching her,
> and sometimes holding my hands a few inches above her spine . . .
> Our contact allowed Barbara to feel more discrete, intricate modalities
> of movement, as well as an abundance of new sensations. Her ability
> to feel herself moving from the inside was a revelation. She told me
> it was the first time she felt herself as whole. In that moment there
> was no paralysis!
>
> (1997: 68)

The therapy work, combined with hours of practice by Barbara on her own, led to increased movement and freedom of breath:

> It was about a year into our process that her knees began to move –
> micro-movements encircling her entire knee area. A micro-movement
> resembles a subatomic pulsation of light, the smallest visible bit of
> movement. Seemingly, they emerged from a deep source, modulating
> the skin and leaving it iridescent . . . I saw small quivers permeating
> her calf. Deep inside sparked the electrical currents of life.
>
> (1997: 70)

Barbara's pelvis, legs and even her feet began to become able to make small movements. However:

> Barbara's original injury was overlaid by years of compensation.
> This presented a complex problem. We were basically dealing with
> two levels of stasis, one traumatic, the other habitual. Unchanging
> compensation can be viewed as another form of paralysis.
>
> (1997: 68–9)

At this stage a more explicitly *psycho*therapeutic encounter became necessary:

> Other aspects of Barbara's paralysis became evident. Her defenses
> were dissolving and revealing a core of self-hatred and despair . . .
> As I became more involved with her life, I grasped more fully the
> undercurrents of her despair, her emotional storms, her wheelchair-
> bound identity, and her social isolation. From my perspective, the
> injury was not localized in her spine, but spread everywhere, reaching
> out in many directions. Her attention, however, was perpetually
> riveted on her legs, as if by sheer concentration she could force
> them to walk.
>
> (1997: 70–1)

Barbara's *character* gradually emerged as a major obstacle to healing – in particular, her lifelong tendency to try, to push, to effort: 'The problem ... was to keep her approach to healing from getting too dry and *locked in*. . . . At some point the focused intensity could become constraining, the goal overbearing. Barbara's commitment, though certainly impressive, could become a trap' (Conrad Da'oud 1997: 73).

In fact, through treating her paralysis issues emerged for Barbara which at some stage become central in most body psychotherapy – issues of surrender:

> As an athlete, Barbara had learnt that forcing was a 'good' thing – her will was indomitable, her commitment enormous, her courage unquestionable ... What I was asking for seemed terrifying; in her mind it meant surrendering to death. . . . For me, this issue was as crucial as achieving wave movements in her diaphragm. I had to keep with her moment to moment, breath to breath, coaxing her away from her ingrained habit. A molting process appeared to be taking place in which the web of old values could be shed.
>
> (1997: 75–6)

At this stage, perhaps unsurprisingly, issues of sexuality and sensuality began to emerge. This was particularly charged for Barbara because her original accident had occurred when she was 18 years old and on her way to an illicit weekend with her boyfriend: 'Barbara's driving urgency left little room to register the undulating lushness taking place inside of her. . . . Sexuality was the betrayer – got her into trouble – was too frightening. Confusion nestled below her hips. . . . By slowing down she began to register sensual feelings by degrees' (Conrad Da'oud 1997: 76).

A healing crisis developed, of a kind by no means restricted to those with overt paralysis: 'We entered the Forbidden City. As Barbara permitted herself more feeling without demand, the level of her self-hatred was increasingly revealed. The room would grow thick with shame and disgust. She would work herself into emotional storms that vibrated the rafters' (1997: 76).

Through persistent, sensitive challenge and support, Barbara was slowly able to weather the storm, to 'allow these exquisite feelings to flood her without imposing purposes and conditions on them'. After two decades of work with Conrad Da'oud, in 1996 Barbara no longer qualified as a paraplegic. Although not quite able to walk, 'she has flexion in all her joints, she has quadricep articulation, and she has continuing strength and innovation in her legs, ankles and feet' (1997: 78). Barbara has become an artist and leads movement groups; she lives with a life partner.

Although Conrad Da'oud has some specific skills not shared by other body psychotherapists, her work shows well the required combination of bodily and psychological sensitivity – indeed, how these 'two' elements are for the body psychotherapist actually one. Her ability to generate rich imagery for the therapeutic process is not only useful for telling the story, but also an essential element in that process. It is part of the magical, shamanic side of body psychotherapy which has existed from its beginnings. Wilhelm Reich, whose own perceptions of bodily patterns were extremely vivid, used to think about his clients through the medium of totemic animals:

> The total expression of the body can usually be condensed in a word or formula which, sooner or later in the course of the character-analytic treatment, suggests itself. Strangely enough, they are usually formulas and names derived from the animal kingdom, such as 'fox', 'pig', 'snake', 'worm', etc.
>
> (Reich [1942] 1983: 302)

Goals, applicability and contraindications

Looking through the stories of clients, practitioners and imaginary sessions in this chapter, we can identify some goals which seem to feature in body psychotherapy. The overarching goal, for many body psychotherapists as well as other sorts of therapists, is clearly to follow and support the client's process; or, put in more ordinary language, to work out what is trying to happen and help it to happen. Many of the specific interventions and activities are actually with this intention. There are also some general ideas and beliefs common in body psychotherapy that certainly influence the sort of *outcome* which practitioners are hoping for. Often they will hope to get there by supporting the client's process, rather than by any specific input of their own. But the outcome picture held by the practitioner seems bound to influence the shape of the work, if not directly then indirectly.

Many, though by no means all, body psychotherapists work with some concept of somatic memory (Van der Kolk 1994); the idea that, as Reich put it, 'every muscular rigidity' – or, indeed, every other bodily restriction – 'contains the history and meaning of its origin' (Reich [1942] 1983: 300); and that by releasing the restriction and reowning the memory, most importantly the emotional memory, a person can dissolve a corresponding pattern of psychological constraint. We shall look at various theoretical formulations of this idea later on. Hence, body psychotherapists will tend in practice to encourage and support spontaneous bodily impulses and experiences, in the expectation that these will lead to some form of completion, re-enactment and/or discharge. Many body psychotherapists work with some conception of *character* – a name for the larger pattern of psychosomatic holdings which in part define each individual: what Richard Strozzi Heckler calls our 'conditioned tendency' (1984: 19ff).

This is why body psychotherapists will often encourage clients to stay with and fully experience unpleasant, painful bodily states. But they are also interested in positive, pleasurable states. As Dean Juhane says – of bodywork rather than body psychotherapy, but the two are closely linked – it seeks to produce 'the displacing of the patient's focus from his body as a source of pain to his body as a source of pleasure and comfort, the physical relaxation which diminishes emotional anxiety, and the restoration of the possibility of control over the situation' (1987: 333). Body psychotherapy has many ways, some of which we will explore, of describing a state of pleasurable, focused aliveness which grows out of the ground of the body. One of its goals is to encourage and foster this state in its clients.

Body psychotherapists pretty much universally believe that it is a good thing for people to relate positively to their body – to listen to it, to identify with it ('I am a body' rather than 'I have a body'), to respect its needs and desires. Many of them believe that this is not generally how things are in our society: that 'the entire structure of our society runs counter to this way of life' (Heckler 1984: 137); that we are trained to devalue and misuse our bodies in a range of ways. As Richard Grossinger forcefully expresses it: 'The majority treat their body like a date picked up at the singles bar. They hustle it, punish it, and try to make it give them things they want' (1995, Vol. 1: 41).

This attitude – in effect, seeing the body as an oppressed and marginalized minority – links body psychotherapy to a broader social tendency, one which embraces the Green movement, much New Age and New Paradigm thinking, and a general critique of global capitalism and its values. At the same time, some of the body psychotherapy scene can be linked to a consumerism of all things beautiful, including beautiful bodies, and an implicit avoidance and denial of difficulty, pain and struggle.

My central point, though, is that beyond the specific benefits which body psychotherapists see in their clients 'listening to the body' – for example, the alleviation of physical or psychological symptoms – there is a wider programme of facilitating a fundamental change in how we all experience our bodies. Reich summed up this goal in his constant use of the word 'surrender'. In his view, we need to recognize the greater wisdom of our somatic aspect over our mental aspect and to let our bodies lead the dance between the two. He connected this directly with our capacity to surrender to the experience of orgasm, and hence to pleasure and relaxation in general, of which orgasm was for Reich the archetype. A similar attitude comes over clearly in Conrad Da'oud's account, though she is not a Reichian as such.

Although body psychotherapists vary in the centrality that they give to sexual expression, most of them agree with Reich's view that our body experience is our main potential source of security, self-confidence and wisdom; and that body psychotherapy can and should repair the balance between our somatic and psychic aspects. In Freudian terms this corresponds to rebalancing the id and the ego, so that the ego/mind recognizes its own limitations and its ultimate dependence on the id/body for its ground of being. In more process-centred terms, we are talking about rebalancing the relationship between 'state' and 'process', so that the individual is able to become more flexible and open to new experience. The Gestalt therapist Barry Stevens talks about 'decontrolling' our bodies: 'Learning how to decontrol my body – not just "relaxation" – is one of the ways of arriving at some understanding of natural functioning and getting in touch with how I interfere with it' (1977: 160).

If this is the healing project of body psychotherapy, the proposed outcome on which its techniques are based, then for whom is it likely to be useful? While body psychotherapy is ready and willing to work with most client groups, it is perhaps especially appropriate for two groups: those whose primary experience is already bodily, proprioceptive – people who 'live in their bodies' – and whom the therapist must meet there if useful work is to take place; and, on the other hand, those who 'live in their heads', whose primary experience is mental, cognitive – and whose bodies are crying out to be recognized and valued and communicated with. Clearly these two groups must be approached very differently (and many in the second group may shy away from it), but body psychotherapy offers a particular gift to each.

Like most intensive therapies, body psychotherapy is perhaps contraindicated for people in a state of psychosis or near-psychosis, for whom the increase of charge which it facilitates might be overwhelming. Having said that, however, skilled body practitioners may be able to 'titrate' the increased charge while working to strengthen the client's defences and their ability to manage stimuli (Levine 1997; Rothschild 2000). Reich wrote an extensive case history of work along these lines with a schizophrenic client (Reich [1950] 1972: 399ff). Similarly, it is often said that bodywork would be unsuitable for abuse survivors, since it would tend to retraumatize them. Again, this may apply only to unskilled body psychotherapy and there are several recent approaches specifically aimed at post traumatic stress disorder (PTSD), including abuse survivors (see Chapter 4).

Overall, then, perhaps we can only say that body psychotherapy is potentially of benefit to all or most people under the right circumstances; but of course the most crucial of those circumstances is that the person is open to experiencing body psychotherapy. This depends partly on where the individual has got to in their life, but also on the availability of skilled body therapy, and of information about the point and purpose of that therapy. This book is intended as a contribution to that end.

CHAPTER 2

Foundations of body psychotherapy

To write about the body is not to theorize abstractly: it is to join fates with other bodies.

(Frank 1998: 229)

We now have something of a change of pace. The previous chapter was, possibly, emotionally demanding. This next one may be intellectually demanding. It examines the theoretical basis of body psychotherapy; if you like, its world view and the sources of that world view. As with most therapies, however – in fact, as with most human enterprises – that world view is often not conscious and available for inspection. Many body psychotherapists could tell you little about the origins or theoretical basis of their work. So this chapter is as much a resource for practitioners themselves as for those coming fresh to the subject. The first task is to reach a definition and description of body psychotherapy itself. As we shall see, this is not a straightforward task.

Again, as with Chapter 1, I want to alert you to your somatic reactions (and to encourage you to bear this in mind throughout the whole book). You have had a chance in the first chapter to notice how your embodied self reacts to reading about some emotionally charged material. Now you have an opportunity to notice how you react to material which, while it does have considerable emotional meaning, is largely couched in intellectual and abstract terminology. What differences are you aware of in your embodied response as you read Chapter 2? Does your body get bored and 'go to sleep', or become agitated; or does it have a sufficiently good relationship with your mind to be able to absorb intellectual food?

Body psychotherapy and bodywork: embodied relationship

The strongest umbrella organization in the field, the European Association for Body Psychotherapy (EABP), defines body psychotherapy as follows:

> A distinct branch of Psychotherapy, well within the main body of Psychotherapy, which . . . involves a different and explicit theory of mind–body functioning which takes into account the complexity of the intersections and interactions between the body and the mind. The common underlying assumption is that the body is the whole person and there is a functional unity between mind and body. . . . Many other approaches in Psychotherapy touch on this area. Body-Psychotherapy considers this fundamental.
>
> (EABP website, see Appendix)

It goes on to say that a body psychotherapist 'works with the person as an essential embodiment of mental, emotional, social and spiritual life. He/she encourages both internal self-regulative processes and the accurate perception of external reality'.

In this book, we shall consider all of the points made in this definition, what they mean, and what theoretical and research-based support exists for them. We should observe that the EABP definition draws a strong distinction between *body psychotherapy* on the one hand and *bodywork* on the other:

> There are also a wide variety of techniques used within Body-Psychotherapy and some of these are techniques used on the body involving touch, movement and breathing. There is therefore a link with some Body Therapies, Somatic techniques, and some complementary medical disciplines, but whilst these may also involve touch and movement, they are very distinct from Body-Psychotherapy.
>
> (EABP website)

This is a valid and important point: body psychotherapy and bodywork cannot be equated. Simultaneously, though, we need to recognize the inextinguishable connection between the two – the braided involvement of each with the other, which is at the heart of the historic enterprise of body psychotherapy, giving it, perhaps, its deepest purpose as well as its deepest problems.

By *bodywork* I mean to indicate the whole ensemble of healing practices which work on, with, or through the body (for these distinctions, see Heckler 1984: 15ff; on bodywork, see Grossinger 1995). Some well-known examples – and of course many distinctions could be made between them – are osteopathy, cranio-sacral therapy, physiotherapy, shiatsu,

Rolfing and massage. None of these practices claims to be psychotherapy. However, most or all of them in different ways are based on some idea of body–mind *unity*, of psychosomatic function: the sense, expressed in many different terms, that in working with the body we are working with the mind and in working with the mind we are working with the body. Most or all of them would hence argue that a person's beliefs and feelings manifest in their body and, conversely, that changes in the body can and do facilitate changes in belief and feeling. This is also the fundamental position of body psychotherapy (see the next section of this chapter).

The difference between the two, then, seems to be largely one of training. Body psychotherapists are specifically trained (sometimes self-trained, as with the originators of the field) to work psychotherapeutically through the body. This notion is not without some difficulty, of course: 'psycho-' clearly implies 'to do with the psyche'. However, if we conceive of psyche not as *over and against* soma, but as *complementary* and even in some senses *identical* to it, then the practice of working somatically through the psyche, and psychotherapeutically through the soma, becomes comprehensible (for a psychoanalytic version of these ideas see Winnicott 1949).

Body psychotherapy recognizes that there is no living human body without mind – no soma without psyche; and therefore that in approaching a human body we are also approaching a human mind. Whatever tools and safeguards are appropriate for a verbal approach to therapy are therefore also appropriate – with certain changes – for a bodily approach. This is a key distinction between body psychotherapists and most body-workers. Like other psychotherapists, body psychotherapists recognize and address all the manifold ways in which human beings resist, evade, deny, attack, mutilate, distort and erase deep contact with themselves and each other. They recognize, therefore, that to assume the client wants to co-operate, 'get better', or improve her functioning is frequently a grave error. They recognize the complex pathways of desire.

This does not amount, however, to an easy and absolute distinction between bodywork and body psychotherapy. Many bodyworkers would agree with much or all of the above. A number of them work very skilfully with these sorts of issues and, in addition, many have much greater technical skills with 'the body as body' than the average body psychotherapist. Richard Grossinger says of bodywork in general, not just of body psychotherapy:

Its methods arise from the epistemology and phenomenology of a body and reach beyond the body itself to a body image, an inner body realm, social communication, and space itself. Thus, somatics has more to do with the body experienced from within than the body manipulated from without.

(Grossinger 1995, Vol. 2: 199)

Any practitioner able to subscribe to this sort of understanding is, surely, a body psychotherapist in fact if not in name – though not necessarily a sufficiently skilled one.

Looking from the side of bodywork practice, one can therefore consider body psychotherapy as a logical historical development whereby certain implications and approaches are gradually separated out from the general field of bodywork, and take on a separate identity, represented by a name, by a focused training and by various organizational phenomena. This is the usual way in which new occupations and professions emerge. Individuals and groups develop new practices, local and specific skills emerging from their encounter with particular tasks. These are eventually recognized by themselves and others as new and begin to link up and interact with other parallel developments.

What then are the specific practices of body psychotherapy – the features held in common by the whole ensemble of parallel activities, which have enabled them to recognize and hail each other and form a common identity? I would suggest that the key feature is a conscious focus on *relationship*. The human body is not something that exists on its own, in isolation. As we shall see later, it has an innate, organismic apparatus for forming relationship with others – it *needs* others for its well-being in very fundamental ways. Conversely, we form relationships through and as our bodies, using structures which have evolved for that precise purpose. (All of these issues are discussed at length later in this chapter.)

Psychotherapy as a whole has always, in many of its traditions, focused on the therapeutic relationship as a way of illuminating and affecting the client's style of relating to self and others. It would not be wrong, though perhaps incomplete, to describe psychotherapy as a practice of relating. Looking from the side of psychotherapy, therefore, we can see body psychotherapy as an extension of this into a new realm: a practice of *embodied relating*.

An empirical effect of this distinction is that many body psychotherapists, but very few bodyworkers, work entirely verbally with some or many of their clients for some or all of the time. For body psychotherapists the relationship is primary, and directs the technical unfolding of the therapy. For certain clients the body is not an acceptable route for exploring their process. It is too frightening, or too alien, or too 'irrelevant'; or they cannot yet feel enough trust for their therapist to enter this area of experience; or they sexualize relationship through the body. Bodyworkers, generally speaking, assume that their clients have come to work with and through the body. The body psychotherapist, generally speaking, does not. However, she will probably feel that, whatever the client's choices, *she* is still working through the body, if only her own. To bring our own body to the therapeutic relationship may be the most fundamental move of body psychotherapy.

From this point of view, 'body psychotherapy' may be better under-stood as 'holistic psychotherapy' or 'bodymind psychotherapy'; with most existing mainstream practices redescribed as 'verbal psychotherapy' (only). From this perspective, body psychotherapy is a name only for the most unusual and unfamiliar aspects of the practitioner's activity – certainly not for all of it. It may turn out that the professional body psychotherapy organizations have made an error in accepting and adopting this limiting label for what they do (Totton 2002b: 203); although, of course, names can come to denote something very different from their literal meaning.

Body psychotherapy, then, is a therapy for the whole person which approaches whatever facet of a given individual – body symptoms, sensa-tions, feelings, images, thoughts, subtle energy, spirituality – is most accessible in this moment as a way of making contact. It then tries to work inwards from that point to the more defended, ignored or excluded aspects of that person's being. It is body psychotherapy only in that it does not *exclude* the body, but treats embodiment as an intrinsic and important feature of human existence.

This raises the question: Can body(mind) psychotherapy take over conventional verbal models of clinical practice and modify them for its own use, as some practitioners are trying to do; or is there the possibility, or necessity, of unique body(mind) psychotherapy models and theories? It will take several more chapters before we are able to reach some answers to this question.

History

> The unconscious does not merely reveal itself in dreams, it reveals itself in every gesture, in the twitching of the forehead, the beating of the heart, yet also in the quiet warning of a uric-acid diathesis.
> (Groddeck [1917] 1977a: 116)

In Chapter 4 we will be surveying the main styles of body psychotherapy existing today. The aim of this current section is to provide a brief historical context, a picture of the lines of influence and argument, which should be of use in understanding the rest of this chapter and Chapter 3. This task is made more complex by the way in which the core themes of body psychotherapy are independently rediscovered over and over again, both consciously and unconsciously. For example, Anton Mesmer, Georg Groddeck, Arnold Mindell and Stanislaf Grof have each independently developed their own forms of body psychotherapy, ap-parently without drawing on the main line of development from Freud through Reich (Mesmer, of course, preceded Freud by a century).

To go further afield, Ots (1994) describes the recent emergence in China of new *qigong* (Chi Kung) forms known as *zifa donggong*, '*qigong* of spontaneous movements'. These forms encourage participants to surrender to movements and vocal sounds, to 'shake their hands and limbs, the head or even the whole body . . . shout, scream, laugh or cry, touch or embrace others, etc.' (Ots 1994: 122). This work is to some extent underground and little discussed; it clearly involves an experience of releasing old buried emotions, as in body psychotherapy (Ots 1994: 127). The history of body psychotherapy also involves repeated cross-fertilization with various traditions of bodywork. Examples include Reich drawing from German breathwork and bodywork traditions (Totton 1998: 240); Gerda Boyesen from Norwegian psychiatric physiotherapy; the Lomi School from martial arts; and Rebirthing from Kriya yoga (for these last three, see Chapter 4).

The central figures of explicit, self-identified body psychotherapy, the 'ancestors' of virtually all later practitioners, are Sigmund Freud, Wilhelm Reich, Fritz Perls and (I would argue, rather more controversially than the first three) Arnold Mindell. Carl Jung has also had a surprisingly powerful influence on the field. The obvious fact that all five of these are white males with central European ancestries suggests a certain limitation to the field, which we will look at in Chapter 6. For now, though, I will simply summarize their contributions and influences.

Although the modern psychoanalytic world wholly rejects body psychotherapy, in 1895 Freud himself wrote to Wilhelm Fliess: 'Yesterday Mrs K again sent for me because of cramplike pains in her chest . . . In her case I have invented a strange therapy of my own: I search for sensitive areas, press on them, and thus provoke fits of shaking that free her' (Masson 1985: 120). Freud dropped this 'strange therapy' completely, but psychoanalysis remained *theoretically* engaged with the body, whose 'drives' are the source of our unconscious desire. The rejection of these desires by our conscious awareness – rejection of the 'body' by the 'mind', in effect – is seen as the cause of many ills. Freud was originally a pioneer neuroscientist, and his therapy originated in a failed attempt to create a biologically-based psychology. Lacking the scientific data and vocabulary to achieve this task, he 'metaphorized' his neurology and called it psychoanalysis (Totton 1998).

The body as a *clinical* issue resurfaced in the work of Freud's great follower, Sandor Ferenczi, who developed a form of somatic trauma therapy (Totton 1998: 57–68); and then more systematically and completely through the practitioner generally seen as the founder of body psychotherapy proper, Wilhelm Reich. Both Reich and Ferenczi were strongly influenced by the brilliant maverick analyst Georg Groddeck, who used deep massage in which 'the patient's changing expressions reveal hidden secrets of his soul . . . Unconscious impulses . . . betray themselves in his involuntary movements' (Groddeck [1931] 1977b: 236).

Although Reich was excluded from the International Psychoanalytic Association in 1934 – partly because of his focus on the body (Sharaf

1984: 175–91) – his work and thought remained deeply informed by the themes and issues of Freudian analysis (Totton 1998). However, Reichian therapy was mainly taken up in the context of humanistic psychotherapy and the 'growth movement' of the 1960s and 1970s. Despite the analyst Melanie Klein's deep interest in the body's role in forming our categories of experience (e.g. Klein [1930] 1988, [1933] 1988), the body has been increasingly remote from mainstream psychoanalytic practice. As we shall see in Chapter 4, Reich's heirs have developed his work in many different directions, some continuing the direct physical intervention of his late style, others staying with his earlier, more gentle and subtle approach.

Reichian ideas made a considerable input into the whole group of body therapies which grew up around the idea of 'primal trauma' in the 1960s and 1970s: Arthur Janov's Primal Therapy itself, and its various offshoots, together with other approaches which focus specifically on the trauma of birth. Another form of birth-oriented work with a very different emotional flavour and a more or less independent origin, is Leonard Orr's Rebirthing. This is one of several body therapies, including Reich's own work, which use the breath as a means of focusing and amplifying bodily sensations and impulses. A modern example is Stanislav Grof's Holotropic Breathwork, which parallels many of Reich's later techniques.

Reich also deeply influenced Fritz Perls, the founder of Gestalt Therapy, who was in analysis with Reich. Perls's early book *Ego, Hunger and Aggression* ([1947] 1969) forms a fascinating bridge between Reichian psycho-analysis and Perls's new system. However, Gestalt tends to use bodywork in a very different way from Reichian and neo-Reichian therapies, emphasizing here-and-now, process-centred aspects of bodily experience rather than the ways in which our bodies carry the history of childhood trauma and frustration – the 'how' rather than the 'why' of the client's problems.

This here-and-now focus is, if anything, even more apparent in the other major non-Reichian contemporary therapy which includes the body: Arnold Mindell's Process Oriented Psychology. Mindell was formerly a Jungian analyst and sees Jung as a major source of his approach. There are other Jungian body psychotherapists, drawing on Jung's concept of the 'somatic unconscious' (1947); see for instance Chodorow (1991); McNeely (1987); Schwartz-Salant and Stein (1986). Mindell regards the body as a crucial terrain for 'dreaming', a term which he extends to cover any sort of extra-conscious signals through which our process communicates itself. The parallels of Mindell's techniques with Gestalt are strong, but apparently largely a case of parallel evolution. The most striking difference, at least from Perls himself, is one of mood – Mindell's work is playful, supportive and permissive rather than confrontational.

There are several other independent or semi-independent manifestations of body psychotherapy: most importantly, perhaps, the expressive body therapies – dance movement therapy, which began in the 1940s, and voice work, which has existed in some form since World War I – and

Eugene Gendlin's Focusing. All of these are significant and influential. They are also in many cases less clearly *psycho*therapies, more exclusively body-focused, less likely (except in the case of some dance therapies) to focus on the therapeutic relationship.

All of the forms of work discussed in this section, together with several others, will be further described in Chapter 4. For now, equipped with this basic sketch of the sources and range of body psychotherapy, we can begin to look at its sources of support: the concepts and research evidence which underly its clinical practice.

Bodymind: the ground of body psychotherapy

Somaticists address not the body *per se* but the mind in the body and the neural, corporeal aspect of the epiphenomenal mind.
(Grossinger 1995, Vol. 2: 201)

It would be wrong to speak of the 'transfer' of physiological concepts to the psychic sphere, for what we have in mind is not an analogy but a real identity: the unity of psychic and somatic function.
(Reich [1945] 1972: 340)

At the heart of most forms of body psychotherapy is an awareness of what we can call 'body–mind holism' (or 'wholism'; both words have the same meaning). In contradiction to mainstream western thinking since at least the sixteenth century, body psychotherapy asserts that Descartes was wrong: I do not exist because I think, but because I am embodied. The subject of body psychotherapy is neither the mind alone, nor the body alone, nor even the two linked or in parallel – but the *bodymind*, a unity of which 'body' and 'mind' are each partial facets.

Although this is still a minority position, body psychotherapists are by no means alone in maintaining it. There is an increasing groundswell of belief in our culture that the splitting of body and mind is both non-sensical and damaging. Until recently, this belief existed mainly as a form of mysticism (and was supported by parallel eastern spiritual teachings); but from the middle of the twentieth century, philosophers and scientists have increasingly come together to criticize the body–mind split (for example, Berman 1990; Varela et al. 1992; Young 1994). An important innovator here was Gregory Bateson (1973, 1980), one of the creators of information theory, who argued cogently that 'mental process is always a function of interaction between parts' (1980: 103); and that the human mind is thus located in the interaction of brain, body and environment, all three being essential elements.

This idea has recently been given powerful scientific support by the neuroscientist Anthony Damasio, who believes that 'mind is probably not conceivable without some sort of embodiment' (1994: 234). In close parallel to Bateson, Damasio's picture of the brain is that:

> Neural circuits represent the organism continuously, as it is perturbed by stimuli from the physical and sociocultural environments, and as it acts on those environments. If the basic topic of these representations were not an organism anchored in the body, we might have some form of mind, but I doubt that it would be the mind we do have.
>
> (Damasio 1994: 226)

Damasio suggests that: 'The representations your brain constructs to describe a situation, and the movements formulated as response to a situation, depend on mutual brain–body interactions' (1994: 228). The traditional view has in effect assumed a parallel between the philosophical opposition of 'mind' and 'body', and the physical opposition of 'brain' and 'body'. Damasio makes it plain that neither of these oppositions are tenable – because 'mind' depends on a continuous dialectic of brain and body, as in turn does our perception of our environment:

> To ensure body survival as effectively as possible, nature . . . stumbled on a highly effective solution: *representing the outside world in terms of the modifications it causes in the body proper*, that is, representing the environment by modifying the primordial representations of the body proper whenever an interaction between organism and environment takes place.
>
> (Damasio 1994: 230; original italics)

It is through a shifting and updating 'map' of the state of our whole body that the brain maintains its awareness of the environment – and also our self-awareness. For Damasio, consciousness itself is the 'mapping of the map' of our bodily state. Hence it makes sense to say, echoing Winnicott's 'there is no such thing as a baby', that 'there is no such thing as a brain' – *on its own* (Carroll 2002b). The brain is actually a part of the body, the part that specializes in modelling and representing other parts and the bodymind as a whole. We need our body to think with (Totton 1998: 142ff).

The same conclusion has been reached from a very different angle by Candace Pert, whose research on neuropeptides has uncovered a distributed network throughout the brain and body, weaving brain, endocrine and immune systems into a single whole:

> Neuropeptides and their receptors are a key to understanding how body and mind are interconnected and how emotions can be manifested throughout the body. Indeed, the more we know about neuropeptides, the harder it is to think in traditional terms of a

mind and a body. It makes more and more sense to speak of a single integrated entity, a 'body–mind.'

(Pert 1986: 9)

This realization casts a critical light on the axiomatic opposition be-tween, on the one hand, the central nervous system (CNS), including the brain and the nerves controlling movement, and on the other the autonomic nervous system (ANS), including the nerves controlling the viscera. The convention is to think of these two systems as a pair of opposites, similar to – in some ways identified with – mind/body or brain/body. Yet in more contemporary perspectives, the ANS 'is in no sense functionally separate from the central nervous system, but receiv-ing axons from cells within that system, forms one of the routes by which the central nervous system controls the tissues of the body' (Romanes 1978: 775).

We shall soon see that this 'control' works in both directions. As Juhane reminds us: ' "autonomic", after all, simply means "self-governing". *Which* self is the question at hand' (1987: 295; original italics).

A host of neuroscientists, psychologists, developmental specialists and other have united to offer support for the basic concept of the functional identity of mind and body (see, for example, Fogel 1993; Gibson 1979, 1987; Stern 1985; Taylor 1992). Philosophers have begun to join in. George Lakoff and Mark Johnson, in a series of groundbreaking books (Johnson 1987; Lakoff 1987; Lakoff and Johnson 1980), have developed an account of language and cognition which is anchored firmly in the body. They argue (in parallel to Melanie Klein, although she never fully spells this out) that our whole conceptual framework is necessarily built up in a series of bodily *metaphors*, at a pre-verbal as much as at a verbal level.

By this they mean a lot more than the often-repeated list of body-based images for psychological states – 'stiff-necked', 'gut feeling', 'leaves a bad taste', and so on. They are referring to the primary categories from which our conceptualization is built – categories like 'in', 'out', 'up', 'down', 'through'. In *Philosophy in the Flesh* (1999) Lakoff and Johnson deconstruct and strip away the traditional western concept of 'Dis-embodied Reason', to reveal the 'Embodied Person':

> Our conceptual system is grounded in, neurally makes use of, and is crucially shaped by our perceptual and motor systems. . . . We can only form concepts through the body. Therefore, every understand-ing we have of the world, ourselves, and others can only be framed in terms of concepts shaped by our bodies. . . . Because concepts and reason both derive from, and make use of, the sensorimotor system, the mind is not separate from or independent of the body.
>
> (Lakoff and Johnson 1999: 555)

Parallel ideas have been put forward by Maxine Sheets-Johnstone in *The Roots of Thinking* (1990), where she uses a phenomenological account of hominid evolution to argue that 'thinking is modeled on the body' (1990: 5) and that 'concepts fundamental to human life originated and originate in animate form and the tactile-kinesthetic body' (7). For example, she relates tool-making to the experiential qualities of teeth (1990: 28ff), and our grasp of number to the binary function of the body – left-right, front-back, etc. – inherent in our upright posture (1990: 71ff). Other phenomenologists have also contributed to an account of embodiment, beginning with Merleau-Ponty (Cataldi 1993) and including in particular Elizabeth Behnke (1995, 1997).

All of this puts in question traditional oppositions between different levels of the 'body–mind hierarchy'; for example, the idea that a problem is *either* psychological *or* neurological *or* biochemical *or* . . . Every bodymind state is all of these and there is little value in constructing causal chains to determine which is the most 'fundamental'. Instead we should ask which perspective is most interesting or most useful in a given situation. This has important clinical implications. As I have written elsewhere:

> A physiological or biochemical interpretation of emotional distress involves closing one's eyes and ears to the greater part of human experience – like someone who insists that love is just a matter of glandular secretions. . . . Psychoactive drugs may well be indicated in emergency situations; but drugs can no more remedy our psychological difficulties than they can teach us mathematics, render us witty, or turn us into Buddhists.
>
> (Totton 2000: 110–11)

Understanding the bodymind

> The self's most basic foundations are in systems that represent the body.
>
> (Carroll 2001)

> Our legs and arms are full of torpid memories.
>
> (Proust 2000: 9)

As we have just seen, body psychotherapy looks to many other fields of study for its theoretical framework and research support, including philosophy, psychology, psychoanalytic theory, biochemistry, biophysics, physiology, anatomy and, perhaps most importantly, neuroscience. In what follows, my central focus will be neuroscientific evidence and theory, but I will also draw on relevant material from other disciplines.

'Neuroscience' is the currently used term for the whole multi-aspected scientific discipline which investigates the nervous system, including the brain. Ever since Reich's research on the autonomic nervous system in the 1930s, body psychotherapy has tended to draw on contemporary work in neuroscience (as did Freud in his formulation of psychoanalysis). However, the field has changed and developed so fast – and never more so than at the present – that any conclusions reached must necessarily be tentative and provisional. Different schools and authors have often each taken up one particular segment of neuroscientific research and developed it as the entire basis for their theory.

Part of the reason for this – apart from the sheer difficulty of comprehending the whole of this vast field – is that most body psychotherapists have from the start been trawling for material which will support their pre-existing experience and intuition. Probably no one has studied neuroscience in order to work out from scratch how to conduct body psychotherapy. Very properly, practitioners who often have great knowledge of what works in practice have looked to neuroscience for some explanation of why that might be the case; and this explanation has in turn, of course, generated new ideas about practice. However, neuroscience is such a fluid and creative field at the moment that it is not hard to 'cherry-pick' research findings to support a wide range of different theories.

Despite this danger, there is a tremendous amount of potential input from contemporary neuroscience into psychotherapy in general, and body psychotherapy in particular – the latter, because neuroscience is producing a great deal of material about what we have been calling embodiment. From the wealth of recent findings, I am going to focus on four particularly relevant areas, all four of which overlap and interact: emotion, socialization, trauma, and memory.

Emotion

It has been apparent at least since Freud – himself an early neuroscientist, whose insights are now being rehabilitated (Schore 1994; Solms and Turnbull 2002; Totton 1998) – that emotion (often referred to by both psychoanalysts and neuroscientists as 'affect') is a form of experience which transgresses the supposed 'mind/body boundary'. Our feelings are both *mental* and, as the other sense of the word 'feel' indicates, *somatic*. Hence there is now evidence that at least the negative emotions – anger, disgust, fear and sadness – can be differentiated physiologically (Berkowitz 1999); and that these differences correspond with our internal perceptions of these feelings, for example:

> Felt heat seems to be an important aspect of many people's mental representation of anger. . . . The prevailing metaphor in the public's

conception of anger is that of a hot liquid in a closed container, as when we say an angry person is 'hot under the collar' or 'all steamed up'. . . . Taken together, the findings are consistent with the marked dilation of the blood vessels and heightened stimulation of the voluntary muscles.

(Berkowitz 1999: 412)

Some researchers have gone further in seeking to derive our emotions, in their full psychosocial complexity, from original physiological sources:

We propose that disgust originated in the widespread distaste/oral rejection response seen in many mammals in response to certain categories of tastes, e.g. bitter tastes, and that the output side of this disgust program was appropriated by a wide range of elicitors, appraisals and meanings. We trace a trajectory from animal disgust origins centered on food selection and protecting the body from harmful ingestants to ideational disgust serving to protect the soul from harmful influences. Disgust expands from 'out of mouth' to 'out of mind'.

(Rozin et al. 1999: 431)

These authors go on to argue that 'disgust becomes a major, if not *the* major force for negative socialization in children' (1999: 439).

The growing field of 'affective neuroscience' (Panksepp 1998; Schore 1994) is showing us the central role of embodied emotion in establishing and maintaining our sense of self and self-value. Emotions are seen as the most complex expression of the processes by which our organism self-regulates (Damasio 2000) – in effect, the language in which our bodymind speaks to itself. As Trevarthen puts it, 'emotions hold the self together' (Trevarthen 2001). Schore argues that 'the regulation of affect is a central organizing principle of human development and motivation' (Schore 2001b: 9–10).

At the same time, affect is more and more deeply understood as a complex neurological phenomenon – one which, just as it philosophically marries mind and body, neurologically marries the CNS and ANS, the voluntary and involuntary aspects of our embodiment.

Emotion depends on the communication between the autonomic nervous system and the brain; visceral afferents convey information on physiological state to the brain and are critical to the sensory or psychological experience of emotion, and cranial nerves and the sympathetic nervous system are outputs from the brain that provide somatomotor and visceromotor control of the expression of emotion.

(Porges 1997: 65)

In other words, affect as a concept and as a phenomenon dissolves the rigid distinction between brain and body, central nervous system and autonomic nervous system: 'the key to understanding the cerebral cortex, then, appears to be the body' (Neafsey 1990: 147).

Socialization

Contemporary neuroscience rehabilitates feeling – conventionally believed to be an obstacle to rationality – as an efficient and high-speed way of processing and evaluating data (Panksepp 1998; Schore 1994). This is particularly true for social interaction, where emotions act as both a means of appraisal – 'Is this person friend or foe?' – a means of feedback – 'I like you/don't like you' – and a cue to action – for example, coming closer or going away. Hence there is a strong case for believing that emotion occurs 'in the context of evolved systems for the mutual regulation of behavior, often involving bodily changes that act as signals' (Brothers 1997: 123). As Trevarthen says, writing from an infant development perspective: 'The emotions constitute a time–space field of intrinsic brain states of mental and behavioral vitality that are signaled for communication to other subjects and that are open to immediate influence from the signals of these others' (1993: 155).

Brothers puts it succinctly: 'Emotion cannot be defined with reference to the mind or body of only one animal or person' (1997: 123). Hence arises the new field of 'social neuroscience' (Cacioppo et al. 1996): the study of bodies in relationship, of how our capacity for and style of relating to others is created and mediated through neurological systems – and, at the same time, how our neurology is created and mediated through relationship. This offers support not only for specific approaches to body psychotherapy, but also for its very existence, as a practice of embodied relating.

Much of this data derives from the study of infant–carer interactions, where the fact that emotional expression is 'hard-wired' into the human face (Ekman 1973, 1999) and the human voice (Kitamura and Burnham 1998) is of crucial importance. Vital development occurs through facial and vocal mirroring between baby and – usually – mother (Heimann 1991; Meltzoff and Moore 1989, 1997).

Stern's work on 'affect attunement' between infant and carer (Stern 1985: 138–61) shows the crucial role of affect in general in the development of core identity, because of the stable feedback that emotional expression gives the infant: 'The constellation of three different kinds of feedback: from the infant's face [i.e. proprioceptive sensation], from the activation profile, and from the quality of subjective feeling' (Stern 1985: 90). In other words, the 'hardwired', biologically given, cross-culturally stable correspondence of particular internal experience to particular physiognomic expressions helps the infant build up a felt sense of 'this is me'. While intentional facial expressions are activated through the central nervous system, spontaneous emotional expression seems to be activated subcortically (Damasio 1994: 140–2) – or, to put it more simply, authentic expression is beyond conscious control and hence offers a direct correlation with authentic feeling.

Many neuroscientists have come to the realization that emotional interactions during infancy play a critical role in the development of physical, neurological systems for the lifelong preconscious processing of 'socioemotional' information, and for the lifelong capacity to feel stable and secure:

> It is now clear that the development of the critical capacity to create and maintain an internal sense of emotional security comes from the inner, not necessarily conscious knowledge that during times of stress, one can cope, either by autoregulation or going to others for interactive regulation. Developmental psychology and neuroscience are now converging to show that this adaptive ability is essentially established in the three first years of human life, and that it is the product of our early attachments.
>
> (Schore 2001a: 4)

Trauma

This concept underlines the key role of trauma in establishing dysfunctional patterns of experiencing and relating. There are specific developmental windows of opportunity for what Schore calls 'the primary caregiver's psychobiological regulation of the infant's maturing limbic system, the brain areas specialized for adapting to a rapidly changing environment' (Schore 2001b: 7). If we miss these launch windows, then certain capacities may never get into orbit – or not without a great deal of later reparative work. The infant experience around attachment, Schore argues, 'can either positively or negatively influence the maturation of brain structure, and therefore, the psychological development of the infant' (2001b: 9). In a linked paper, Schore offers:

> thoughts on the negative impact of traumatic attachments on brain development and infant mental health, the neurobiology of infant trauma, the neuropsychology of a disorganized/disoriented attachment pattern associated with abuse and neglect, trauma-induced impairments of a regulatory system in the orbitofrontal cortex, the links between orbitofrontal dysfunction and a predisposition to posttraumatic stress disorders, the neurobiology of the dissociative

defense, the etiology of dissociation and body–mind psychopathology, the effects of early relational trauma on enduring right hemispheric function, and some implications for models of early intervention. These findings suggest direct connections between traumatic attachment, inefficient right brain regulatory functions, and both maladaptive infant and adult mental health.

(Schore 2001c: 201)

A series of papers by Bruce Perry and his associates gives a compelling picture of how 'the brain's exquisite sensitivity to experience in early childhood allows traumatic experiences during infancy and childhood to impact all future emotional, behavioral, cognitive, social, and physiologic functioning' (Perry and Pollard 1998). Perry and his co-writers argue that conditions of dramatic change in the childhood environment activate special neurological stress-response mechanisms – primarily connected with the sympathetic nervous system – to promote adaptive survival and a later return to homeostasis. 'Severe, unpredictable, prolonged, or chronic' stress can overwhelm these mechanisms, so that rather than returning to the previous base state, a 'new but less flexible state of equilibrium' is created (Perry and Pollard 1998: 35–6).

This new base state will tend to involve 'hypervigilance, increased muscle tone, a focus on threat-related cues (typically non-verbal), anxiety, behavioral impulsivity' (Perry and Marcellus 1997: 3) – in other words, bodymind traits which are valuable in a situation of immediate threat, but destructive as a permanent state. As well as this 'hyperarousal continuum', some traumatized children show a 'dissociative continuum' response (Perry et al. 1995: 279–82), a tendency to cognitively and/or physically freeze, and often to dissociate in pattern of 'numbing, compliance, avoidance, and restricted affect' (281).

Body psychotherapists frequently encounter the traces of both these patterns in their clients: the individual who cannot relax but is locked into cycles of anxiety and tension, or the individual who seems to be not really 'there', not identified with their here-and-now bodily experience. The assumption, out of the psychotherapeutic tradition originating with Freud, is that these states have to do with early experience. This assumption has now been strongly validated by neuroscientific research, which also offers important pointers on how such problems can be addressed (see the discussion of trauma therapies in Chapter 4).

One perhaps almost universal form of early trauma is touch deprivation. It has been abundantly demonstrated that

Laboratory animals who are given rich tactile experiences in their infancy grow faster, have heavier brains, more highly developed myelin sheaths, bigger nerve cells, more advanced skeletal muscular growth, better coordination, better immunological resistance, more developed pituitary/adrenal activity, earlier puberties, and more active sex lives than their isolated genetic counterparts.

(Juhane 1987: 49)

There is no reason to doubt that the same is true for humans; and also that more complex emotional and social damage is caused by touch deprivation (Montagu 1971) – which as well as being prevalent in many families, is also encouraged or even enforced by many medical regimes around childbirth and childrearing (Prescott 1971).

Memory

How we remember is not yet well understood, but current thinking has some important implications for body psychotherapy. All parts of the brain, it is clear, can store information. Hence we have not only the familiar cognitive memory, but also 'emotional memory' (LeDoux et al. 1990), 'motor vestibular memory' and 'state memory'. Each of these has its own organization and structure and is laid down in different areas of the brain (Perry 1997). In saying this, we need to remember the crucial point made earlier that 'there is no such thing as a brain' – or rather, no point at which we can realistically say that the brain ends and the body begins.

In relation to memory, emotion has the same role that we have discussed elsewhere of providing a qualitative assessment of particular data. It appears likely that: 'Storage of memory for emotionally arousing events is modulated by an endogenous neurobiological system . . . which becomes active in emotionally stressful learning situations, to ensure that the strength of memory for an event is, in general, proportional to its importance' (Cahill 1997: 238).

Emotional memories are stored subcortically, via the amygdala and other related brain areas. As we have seen, 'subcortical' is more or less equivalent to 'bodily'. 'When such memories are established merely by means of subcortical mechanisms, they may be encoded through non-conscious processing and become very resistant to extinction' (Christianson and Engelberg 1999: 217). There is considerable evidence that traumatic memories can be stored, and expressed, unconsciously and non-verbally (Howe et al. 1996; Christianson and Engelberg 1999).

In other words, emotional memories are unconscious – they appear as *feelings*, not as *memories* of feelings – and persistent. There is considerable reason to think that traumatic memories in particular are laid down in such a way as to be highly resistant to extinction, and also hard to bring into consciousness (Cahill 1997; Van der Kolk 1994; vanOyen Witvliet 1997). They are not cognitive in nature, but emotional, motor vestibular and state based. A state (like arousal) can trigger a feeling (like panic);

or conversely a thought (memory of traumatic events) can trigger a subcortical state memory. But of course all these forms of memory are not only, or primarily, traumatic; they are fundamental to our bodymind existence, and, as I have said, essentially non-cognitive.

Motor vestibular memories are the complex bodily skills which we all learn; skills like riding a bicycle or playing a musical instrument, or more fundamentally, walking and talking. These sorts of implicit memory ('implicit' meaning that we cannot examine or discuss them, but only *perform* them) are encoded in body–brain interactions. They cannot be separated out from a person's entire habitual state of embodiment. This is even more true of state memories, which are habitual patterns of bodymind arousal like stress, anxiety or security – the sorts of base states we have already discussed, which are set up often in infancy in response to the environment in which we find ourselves. State memories can often hardly be distinguished from the sorts of functional or physical structures that we have been discussing above, which are either established or not depending on the infant's circumstances. In a sense these memories are just another way of conceptualizing such structures. Any predisposition to respond to a particular cue in a particular way is in essence a memory.

Body psychotherapy clearly accesses motor vestibular and state memories. For example, Perry (1997) suggests that one of the most powerful examples of these is memory related to eating, which can become inextricably associated either with safety, intimacy and nurturing, or with insecurity and emotional disruption. These sorts of memory clusters are the meat and drink – so to speak – of body psychotherapists, the material with which we deal every day. They are the reason why body-oriented practitioners have always thought in terms of 'body memory'. The well-known practitioner Stanley Keleman emphasizes the role of what he calls 'motor memory', arguing that: 'Muscular movement patterns are the source of what we call memory. . . . We recall an actual past muscle pattern together with its emotional associations. By re-experiencing those patterns and associations, we make internal images to represent the event' (Keleman 1987: 28).

All these forms of memory – emotional, motor vestibular and state – are *use dependent*. In other words, they are created and sustained by patterns of activity. Hence, at least in theory, new patterns of memory can change these stubborn unconscious patterns. Juhane (1987: 266ff) discusses motor vestibular memories under the name of 'engrams', and argues that 'counter-productive' and 'traumatic' engrams can be addressed through bodywork:

> Bodywork can be . . . a kind of reverse trauma. By creating through artful manipulation a sustained series of sensory impressions suggestive of pleasure, of softness, of length, of relaxation, the reduced

muscle tone *normally associated with these feelings* can be evoked. And with either local or general reductions of muscle tone comes a veritable parade of sensory effects. . . . All of this constitutes the restoring of the complete and coherent flow of sensory information with which we organize our bodies and our minds.

(Juhane 1987: 275; original italics)

Body psychotherapy, as distinct from bodywork, contributes to this process a deliberate focus on the 'emotional memory' aspects. As Juhane acknowledges, 'my emotions regarding a particular activity . . . *function much like sensory engrams*' (1987: 272; original italics). And emotional memory, in particular, is bound up with the whole of our history of interaction with other people. It is this history which we now need to consider from a bodymind perspective.

The intersubjective bodymind

The social intelligence of the infant is evidently a specific human talent – an inherent, intrinsic, psychobiological capacity that integrates information from many modalities to serve motive states.

(Trevarthen and Aitken 2001: 4)

Research into infant development has established that social interaction begins at or even before birth (for vocal interaction in the womb, see Lecanuet 1996); and that it is as much bodily as mental, 'a fundamentally innate process of *emotional physiology*, by expression of which a primary level of intermental communication is established between human subjects' (Trevarthen and Aitken 2001: 8; my italics).

What Trevarthen and Aitken call the infant's 'primary intersubjectivity' (2001: 5) is a rich bodymind process of 'protoconversation' which they liken to dance and music (6). Like Stern (1985), Trevarthen and Aitken argue that our whole capacity to interact socially and to use language proper is founded on this innate psychobiological skill. However, the infant's communication needs to be elicited and responded to by adults who are capable of expressive tuning in and matching. Trevarthen and Aitken quote research on how infants are affected by postnatal depression:

which causes the mother to express herself without pleasure, with flat affect, and with erratic timing of behaviors that do not engage with the infant's behaviors. . . . Young infants . . . are affected by . . . unsympathetic and inappropriately timed maternal behavior . . . the mother's self-referred, unresponsive state . . . and the quality of speaking that lacks 'musicality' . . . They become distressed and

avoidant and may develop a lasting depressed state that affects communication with persons other than their mother.

(Trevarthen and Aitken 2001: 9)

We must remember, of course, that 'postnatal depression' is not simply
an 'illness', but a complex psychosocial phenomenon at least partly due
to society's expectations of the new mother.

The psychoanalyst Daniel Stern is a leading researcher of infant–carer
attunement (1985; see also Totton 1998). He introduces the helpful concept of 'vitality affect' (Stern 1985: 53–60; cf. Davidson's (1999) work on
'affective style'). Vitality affects are captured by dynamic, kinetic terms
such as 'surging', 'fading away', 'fleeting', 'explosive', 'bursting', 'drawn
out', and so on. For example:

A 'rush' of anger or of joy, a perceived flooding of light, an acceler-
ating sequence of thoughts, an unmeasurable wave of feeling evoked
by music, and a shot of narcotics can all feel like 'rushes'. They all
share similar envelopes of neural firings, although in different parts
of the nervous system. . . . Expressiveness of this kind is . . . inherent
in all behaviour.

(Stern 1985: 54–6)

Stern argues that this sort of quality is primary in the infant's organization of experience. 'Like dance for the adult, the social world experienced by the infant is primarily one of vitality affects' (1985: 57). The
pattern of 'surging', 'bursting', 'explosion' and so on is not tied to any
particular sensory mode, but is abstract, part of the innate capacity for
abstraction which Stern sees as a fundamental building block of infant
experience (1985: 51). This 'abstraction', though, is intrinsically embodied
– the patterns of vitality affect are bodily ones, dances of the flesh.

Stern's description of vitality affects, and of the attunement of carer
and infant through matching vitality affect, illuminates both the theory
and the practice of body psychotherapy. Many texts by body psychotherapists can be read as descriptions of vitality affect, for example this
passage from Wilhelm Reich:

The rhythmicity of one's movements, the alternation of muscular
tension and relaxation in movement, go together with the capacity
for linguistic modulation and general musicality. The sweetness of
children who have not been subject to any severe repressions . . .
has the same basis. On the other hands, people who are physically
stiff, awkward, without rhythm, give us the feeling that they are
also psychically stiff . . . They speak in a monotone and are seldom
musical.

(Reich 1972: 345–6)

Vitality affect provides an empirical foundation for the belief, shared not only by body psychotherapists but by many other practitioners and theorists, that there is a constitutive *bodily* layer of human identity.

The Polyvagal Theory proposed by Stephen Porges (1995, 1997) brings many of the themes we have been examining together with some new ideas. Porges argues that the evolution of the autonomic nervous system (ANS) shows how basic, organismic regulatory affect processes have transmuted into mechanisms of socialization (cf. Trevarthen and Aitken 2001: 21). The Polyvagal Theory links the evolution of the ANS to emotional experience and expression, facial gestures, vocal communication and associated social behaviour:

> Autonomic (visceral) self-preserving and reproductive regulations are elaborated into an emotional signalling mechanism . . . which evolves in the more highly cooperative species into a powerful control of relationships and attachments by negotiatory self-other (complex) emotions.
>
> (Trevarthen and Aitken 2001: 18)

Porges suggests that the autonomic nervous system can best be thought of as consisting of not two divisions, as traditionally, but three: as well as the sympathetic (fight-flight) and parasympathetic (immobilization), he identifies the 'social engagement system', involved with communication – facial expression, vocalization, listening. This system has developed out of one division of the vagus nerve, together with other cranial nerves, 'special visceral efferent pathways' which seem to be neuroanatomically linked with structures that regulate sucking, swallowing and salivation and inhibit our cardiovascular system to calm and soothe us; and also nerves which regulate the muscles of the middle ear and the eyelids, producing a social 'looking and listening' behaviour. (Tensing of middle ear muscles cuts down background noise and amplifies the higher frequencies associated with human voices.)

Porges's theory is exciting because it offers a model of how sophisticated social interaction may have developed directly out of visceral regulation mechanisms, originally concerned with the heart and gut, and still deeply bound up with our capacity to access infant states of calm, soothing feeding. It directly derives our ability to talk from our ability to *suck*, in a style which is very familiar to body psychotherapists. As Porges points out, these systems are related to symptoms experienced by many challenged children including difficulties in listening and making eye contact, highly selective food biases, and behavioural problems like temper tantrums).

The implication of his theory is that the social engagement system is available to us when the environment is perceived as safe. Unsafety and trauma result in the compulsive engagement of the fight/flight (sympathetic) and freezing (parasympathetic) systems, and a perhaps permanent lack of social capacities. A weak social engagement system creates effects like emotional flatness, difficulty in speech recognition and articulation, hypersensitivity to sound and difficult behaviour – all common in children with developmental disorders.

Porges and Bazhenova (n.d.) have made an experimental intervention with a group of autistic children based on the Polyvagal Theory. The children were exposed to a recording of children's songs processed by computer to extract only the frequencies of the human voice. According to the theory, this will stimulate the function of the social engagement system. The small-scale intervention with 40 autistic children had 'immediate and profound effects on behavior . . . many children had dramatic changes in facial affect, spontaneity, listening, communication, and behavioral state regulation'.

Implications

All of this implies that body psychotherapy could play a potentially crucial role in uncovering very fundamental disturbances of embodiment, originating in early childhood, with profound effects on social and emotional functioning and indeed on the individual's sense of self. Body psychotherapy can not only uncover such disturbances but also address them through direct somatic interaction, facilitating a situation in which the individual can develop missing capacities for self-regulation and relationship with others. I would suggest that much of what body psychotherapists instinctively do can be understood within this framework (an extension of the framework offered by Juhane 1987); and conversely, that body psychotherapists can probably improve their effectiveness by including this framework in their awareness.

The assumption of much neuroscience research – reflecting the assumptions of our society – is that this work will ultimately lead to biomedical, technological 'treatments' for early trauma and developmental deficit. Thus Main claims:

> We are now, or will soon be, in a position to begin mapping the relations between individual differences in early attachment experiences and changes in neurochemistry and brain organization. In addition, investigation of physiological 'regulators' associated with infant–caregiver interactions could have far-reaching implications for both clinical assessment and intervention.
>
> (Main 1999: 881–2)

I have tried to show that the real implications of current research are rather different, and in fact more profound: that subtle and powerful modes of 'regulation', 'assessment' and 'intervention' are already inherent in our capacity for embodied relationship, our ability to mutually affect each other's bodymind systems through complex somatic interaction. We don't need to develop a pill, in other words, to heal damage to embodiment, to relationship. No conceivable pill or surgical procedure could facilitate healing more effectively than the skilful use of our embodied humanity in the many forms of body psychotherapy.

Bodymind and society

> We now have the means to exert an unprecedented degree of control over bodies, yet we are also living in an age which has thrown into radical doubt our knowledge of what bodies are and how we should control them.
>
> (Shilling 1993: 3)

It is widely agreed that there has been 'a turn towards the body in contemporary scholarship in the human sciences' (Csordas 1994: xi; cf. Hancock et al. 2000: 10–11). In recent decades an enormous amount of research and writing has taken place on the subject of the body. This no doubt reflects changes in culture itself: 'in conditions of high modernity, there is a tendency for the body to become increasingly central to the modern person's sense of self-identity' (Shilling 1993: 1). Turner argues that we now live in a 'somatic society' (1992: 12), where the body has become 'the principle field of political and cultural activity' (162).

Turning to the body

The body operates as a key nodal point in the complex web of conceptual tensions which make up contemporary thought. Frank suggests that the body is an object of theoretical fascination at the moment because it can be used both as a guarantor of knowledge, something solid to appeal to, and as a demonstration of the many ways in which reality is socially constructed, so that the body is only whatever we (society) make it. Hence there is a creative tension between the body as 'reference point in a world of flux and the epitome of that same flux' (Frank 1991: 40). As Bryan Turner points out, 'the idea that the body is the central metaphor of political and social order is in fact a very general theme in sociology' (Turner 1991: 5; cf. Barkan 1975; Turner 1984). Hence new experiences of the body both derive from new social structures and offer new metaphors for those structures.

According to Lyon and Barbalet, the 'turn to the body' derives from two specifically modern body experiences – the objectified medical body, and the consumerist body: 'The consumerist body is the body we dress, feed and exercise as projects in their own right. This is the body which exists as the body we, but especially others, see' (1994: 51; cf. Featherstone 1991). Sampson (1998: 42–3) also identifies a modern 'turn to the body', but suggests that its sources include feminism (cf. Bayer and Malone 1998: 115), eastern thought, and pentecostalism. There is talk of the 'feminist body' (e.g. Bordo 1993), the 'emotional body' (Freund 1982), the 'social body' (Freund and McGuire 1991), the 'ethical body' (Russell 2000), the 'libidinal body' (Bartky 1988) and many other subspecies of body – a complex terrain on which the 'psychotherapeutic body' jostles for its place!

What relevance does this complex of ideas about the body and culture have for body psychotherapy (which admittedly has so far paid them little attention)? Most centrally, perhaps, they offer an account of 'embodiment as the existential ground of culture and self' (Csordas 1994: 6): a set of ways in which we can think about how the body transmits, encapsulates, indeed bears the brunt of a whole series of social and cultural stresses and tensions – how these are literally *embodied* for the individual, often therefore appearing to her as a basic condition of life, simply the way things are. For example, as Turner describes:

> The 'crisis' in nervous illnesses in the late nineteenth century produced a cluster of conditions – anorexia, agoraphobia, anorexic hysteria, virgin's disease, or various wasting diseases – which can be interpreted as symptomatic of changes in the relationship between the sexes, between public and private space, between the family and the economy within the context of the growing dominance of medicine over moral issues.
>
> (Turner 1991: 23)

This 'cluster of conditions' was the exact ground from which psychoanalysis sprang. But although their sociocultural origins were indeed implied by Freud's theory, the connection was, and remains, easily missed if we hold too narrow a focus on the clinical encounter as something separate from its social context.

Turner offers a relevant context for body psychotherapy in his description of 'three fundamental propositions' inherited by sociology from anthropology:

> First, human embodiment creates a set of constraints . . . but equally important the body is also a potential which can be elaborated by sociocultural development. . . . Secondly, there are certain contradictions between human sexuality and sociocultural requirements. . . . Thirdly, these 'natural' facts are experienced differently according to gender.
>
> (Turner 1991: 4)

We shall look at explicitly political formulations of these issues in the next section.

Emotion and society

Like neuroscience – though, sadly, with as yet very little mutual cross-fertilization – the social sciences have focused recently on the crucial connection between body and emotion, and its role in socialization and social interaction. For example, Lyon and Barbalet identify:

> the crucial role of emotion in the being of the body in society. Our goal has been to develop a framework for seeing the body as agent in, and as locus of intersection of, both an individual psychological order and a social order . . . We have argued that it is through the agency of emotion that this synthesis is accomplished.
>
> (Lyon and Barbalet 1994: 63)

For Burkitt:

> The body and emotion are seen as having pattern and form because they are a part of social relations. These relations, which re-form the body, may not correspond to the prevailing relations of power in society more generally, in which case the body and its habits may appear opposed to the social order. Yet this does not mean it is irrational or pre-social.
>
> (Burkitt 1999: 3)

Burkitt sums up: 'emotions need to be understood as complexes that arise as bodily actions within relations of power and guided by moral precepts' (1999: 6).

The cultural variation in emotional expression is an important theme; for example, Dalgleish points out:

> In many cultures sadness is not considered to be inherently negative, because sadness, or states akin to sadness, are highly valued . . . the variation across cultures in the approach to sadness reflects a culture's view of the perceived lack of self-mastery, and the perceived 'demands' that may thereby be placed on others in the social network as a consequence of sadness. Both lack of self-mastery and demandingness on others are viewed negatively in those cultures which emphasise individuality rather than collectivity and activity rather than passivity.
>
> (Dalgleish 1999: 499)

Hence, Dalgleish argues, sadness can have an important positive social function in that 'it may lead the individual to make emotional and practical demands on others; it can thereby strengthen social bonds' (1999: 499) He also identifies a potential positive function for the individual, in propagating a necessary 'increase in self-focus'.

Body politics

> The appropriation of bodiliness, in all its aspects, from sexuality and reproductive capacities to sensory powers and physical health, strength and appearance, is the fundamental matrix, the material infrastructure, so to speak, of the production of personhood and social identity. What is at stake in the struggle for control of the body, in short, is control of the social relations of personal production. Consistently with this, the body remains the site of some (although by no means all) of the most fundamental forms of social inequality and control in contemporary society. as well as some of its characteristic forms of mystified social consciousness.
>
> (Turner 1994: 28)

If the body is implicated in society and culture, then it is also necessarily implicated in relations of power – the body is political:

> When we say the personal is political, we are suggesting that the body is also politicized. It is the sphere in which consequences of oppression are most easily felt. How an individual experiences his or her body will depend, to a large degree, on the 'others' in the immediate environment, who continuously monitor and interpret his or her bodily processes. To an extent, the body is society's creature. It will live through the image of those who watch, nurture, punish and reward it.
>
> (Brittan and Maynard 1984: 219–20)

Hence what Bourdieu and Wacquant refer to as 'the somatization of social relations of domination' (1992: 172) – the patterns of power and submission in a given society are in effect inscribed on the bodies of its members, through the ways in which they are taught to use and treat their bodies from infancy onwards (Foucault 1977, 1979; Prout 2000).

Riane Eisler restates one of the main themes of the previous section: 'how we image the human body plays a central role in how we image the world' (1996: 163). She goes on to argue:

> How we image the relations between bodies – and most critically, how we experience these relations in our own bodies – is not only a

metaphor for politics in its most basic sense of the way power is defined and exercised. It is how we first unconsciously learn, and continually reenact, the way our human bodies are supposed to relate in all relations, in both what has traditionally been defined as the public and the private spheres.

(Eisler 1996: 164)

Many people – including body psychotherapists from Reich onwards – have long pointed out how western culture has denied and suppressed the body and its needs (e.g. Brown 1968; Reich 1972; Berman 1990; De Meo 1998). The neuropsychologist James Prescott offered some interesting research giving support to Reich's view that the repression of sexuality and the withholding of physical affection in childhood are both socially damaging. He used material on 400 tribal societies to show that 'those societies which give their infants the greatest amount of physical affection were characterized by low theft, low infant physical pain, low religious activity, and negligible or absent killing, mutilating, or torturing of the enemy' (Prescott 1975: 12) and that 'deprivation of body pleasure throughout life – but particularly during the formative periods of infancy, childhood, and adolescence – are very closely related to the amount of warfare and interpersonal violence' (14). These findings dovetail with the neuroscientific reasoning of Schore, Porges and colleagues which we have examined above.

As well as issues of the denial or suppression of the body, however, there are also issues of its exploitation and representation; and these are perhaps even more important in the current phase of our own culture, where there is an explosion of 'repressive desublimation' (Marcuse 1966). To return to Eisler, she puts forward a version of history in which:

the reconceptualization of the female body from a symbol of sexual and spiritual power to an object under the control of men was integral to the prehistoric shift to a dominator social organization ... the bodies of all women, and most men, came to be viewed in terms of the needs and desires of those with the greatest power to hurt, and thus exercise control over, the bodies of others.

(Eisler 1996: 165)

Many feminists and gays, and a much smaller number of straight male gender activists, have identified the body as a key location for political struggle over the definitions of gender and sexuality which are permitted by our society (see, for e.g., Brittan and Maynard 1984; Turner 1994; Davis 1997). From this perspective, every body psychotherapy client presents a body which maps not only the vicissitudes of their personal history, but also the constraints and prohibitions which society imposes on their sex and gender. Problems like anorexia, bulimia, body dysmorphia, impotence and orgastic impotence are only the most obvious effects of this situation.

Like psychotherapy in general, but at an even sharper point, body psychotherapy is faced with the demand that it respond politically – that is, in terms of power relations – to a political situation. Many practitioners are unable or unwilling to make that response. Some operate consciously or, more often, unconsciously from an ideology of sex and gender which seeks to 'help' clients by imposing on them a set of self-understandings which they may experience as wholly alien.

A subtly important way in which gender politics interacts with body psychotherapy is that, in our society, the concept of 'body' is aligned with a number of other important concepts including 'female', 'natural' and 'emotional' (the corresponding opposite set of concepts being, of course, 'mind', 'male', 'cultural' and 'rational'). Not only women, but also other non-mainstream groups in western society, for example, people of colour (middle-class, white males being the mainstream grouping), have tended to be identified with feelings and bodies, and these have been devalued in comparison with mind and reason: 'There is also a politics of emotion. In society's eyes, because we are not all identified with our bodies to the same extent, we are not all regarded as equally emotional. Relations of dominance and subordination can be based on this inequality' (Cataldi 1993: 145).

For many men in particular, identifying with their body and with their emotions feels 'unmanly' in ways which they might find it hard to define. Equally, for many women their alignment with their body and emotions feels like the seal of their oppression. The early body psycho-therapist Wilhelm Reich writes of one male client that when he could finally surrender to his bodily experience 'he was deeply baffled by it. "I would never have thought," he said, "that a man could surrender too." ' (Reich 1983: 328). Partly through our society's coding of gender and sexuality, 'surrender' is identified both with femininity and with subor-dination. Body psychotherapists necessarily have to address these issues in their work.

A related political theme is that already referred to as the 'consumerist body': the body as subject and object of consumption, 'the body we dress, feed and exercise as projects in their own right' (Lyon and Barbalet 1994: 51). As these authors go on to say (summarizing Featherstone 1982): 'In the current configuration of the market economy the body becomes a possession which, through its appearance, provides opportu-nities for social and professional advancement: appearance, display and the management of impression are the capital goods of the consumer economy' (1994: 51). This is equally relevant to the proliferation of gyms and health clubs, or the increasingly urgent need of teenagers and young adults for the right trainers and accessories (an addiction for which some will steal and injure). Lyon and Barbalet point out that the 'consumerist body' has risen as the 'laboring body' has fallen from attention, with the decline in manual labour as a proportion of the workforce. They further emphasize that the consumerist body 'is significantly passive in the way that the laboring body is not . . . as an object of gaze and exchange. The consumerist body is very much the body we have and do things to. In addition . . . the consumerist body is objectified in its relations to others' (1994: 52).

In other words, the consumerist body, in terms of social convention, is feminine. Women tend to bear the brunt of the demands of the consumerist body, which is clearly deleterious in many ways, encouraging us to experience our body as a passive object, almost an 'accessory' itself, something to be exploited just as the natural world is exploited – and also further marginalizing the old, the unattractive, the disabled or unusual looking, who cannot offer a valuable commodity to the market. The consumerist body is a political issue for these reasons, and also because, as Terence Turner reminds us, 'the proliferating commodification of all aspects of bodiliness in contemporary society is driven by the systemic requirements of the accumulation of capital under the specific market conditions of late capitalism' (Turner 1994: 31). In other words, if I treat my body as a commodity, someone can make a buck. The consumerist body, a coming together of profit and misogyny factors, is typified by the Barbie doll, which if life-size would be a mutant with 40-inch breasts, a 22-inch waist, and 5-foot-long legs.

One could use any number of sources to illustrate the role of the consumerist body. In fact, in a break from writing this section, I found an article on the front page of my Sunday newspaper's leisure section entitled 'Oh, You Great Big Beautiful Doll' (Hodge 2002). The subject is Melissa Miller ('Emme'), 'America's most successful "plus size" model':

> By the time I was 12 I was already tall and had developed breasts and hips. Because my stepfather was obese he was very conscious of my [sic!] weight. . . . At home food was always a contentious issue. I was weighed once a week, I was never allowed dessert . . . One day when I was 12, my mother was out and my stepfather got me to undress to my underwear. He took a pen and circled the parts of my body that he thought were problem areas. I was so ashamed, I can definitely say that day marked the beginning of my negative relationship with my body.
>
> (Hodge 2002: 2)

Emme eventually became a successful model, but describes how one photographer 'shouted out in front of everyone, "I am not going to shoot this fattie." ' 'I spent my first big modelling cheque on therapy . . . I felt full of guilt and shame' (Hodge 2002: 2).

Some recent authors have rightly pointed out that power does not run just in one direction, even for the consumerist body. They have emphasized how 'rather than simply adopting versions of femininity that they are invited to emulate, women actively seek to redefine and rearticulate the meaning of these femininities' (Jagger 2000: 56) through the inherent ironization which fashion carries with it; and also the unique capacity of fashion to express intimate bodily pleasures (Cixous 1994). Awareness of this double-edged quality of body consumerism is surely crucial for body-psychotherapeutic work with women. However much fashion can be seen as 'a new way of speaking with the body' (Jagger 2000: 56), this speech still occurs within a regime of objectification.

The body as an object of consumption echoes the body as an object of technological medicine. Modern biomedicine regards the 'body as a machine and . . . the doctor's task as the repair of the machine' (Engel 1977: 131). 'The sick person [becomes] reduced to and understood in terms of the disease that he or she suffer[s] from' (Hughes 1999: 15). And in modern regimes of biomedicine, the subject is enlisted in the surveillance and regulation of her own body and the whole of life takes place in a medicalized space:

> Eating, drinking, sleeping, leisure activities, sexual behaviour, cities and communities have all come under the jurisdiction of medical regulation. The good life has become the healthy life and every one of us is expected to integrate the codes, conduct and prescriptions of such a life into our daily activities.
>
> (Hughes 2000: 19)

Much of this applies also to the equally demanding regimes of complementary medicine and 'self-help'.

Like the consumer body, the medical body is constituted 'objectively' by *vision*, not by *sensation*: hence it is centred externally to itself, in the perception of the other. This is one aspect of what is widely regarded as an hegemonic shift in modern culture towards 'ocularcentrism', the privileging of sight over other senses (Lacan 1977; Levin 1985; Sampson 1998; cf. Cataldi 1993: 146). It implies a corresponding devaluation of proprioception, the internal felt sense of one's own body as process, which is the central subject matter of body psychotherapy. Hence body psychotherapy is directly involved in a multi-faceted cultural struggle over the definition and description of reality: a struggle 'between the *object-body* . . . and *embodiment*' (Sampson 1998: 32).

From Reich onwards, many body psychotherapists have been aware of the political dimensions of their task. As Don Johnson says:

> Underlying the various techniques and schools, one finds a desire to regain an intimate connect with bodily processes: breath, movement

impulses, balance and sensibility. In that shared impulse, this community is best understood within a much broader movement of resistance to the West's long history of denigrating the value of the human body and the natural environment.

(Johnson 1997: xvi)

Grand points out how, just as in other forms of psychotherapy, ignoring the social and political context of one's work can be destructive for the body psychotherapist:

The somatic forming of the sense of self, the complexities of somatic representation of the self and others, are not limited to the caregiver in infancy or to the family of origin.

It is ultimately not useful, for example, to try to explain the hyper-alertness of a young black man in South Central Los Angeles solely on the basis of his early childhood interaction with his caregivers. It is also important to see how representations of gangs, employment opportunity and life expectancy impact the conduct of his flesh.

(Grand 1998: 182)

However, discussion of 'The Body', with that dangerous definite article and implied or actual capitalization, can also take on a distinctly reactionary political tone: an uncontextualized idealization of the body, both by the theoretician – 'we know with our bodies . . . if there is any truth it is the truth of the body' (Game 1991: 192) – and by the body psychotherapist – 'to develop the body's authentic voice, allowing its ancient intelligences to speak forth their wisdom' (Johnson n.d). Such cloudy formulations operate mainly as justifications for whatever the speaker wants to claim as the body's 'truth'.

Conclusion

This chapter has probably been heavy going, and I have deliberately tried to avoid choosing one consistent point of view, taking one side of every argument. The fact is that body psychotherapy finds itself in the middle of a number of shooting wars, and without any conveniently positivistic solid ground on which to stand. The bodymind is in contest, on every level from the political to the metaphysical (which is, of course, itself political), and body psychotherapy least of all can stand aloof from that contest. Each grouping and each practitioner must negotiate this difficult terrain in their own way, forming what alliances they can.

CHAPTER 3

Models, concepts and skills

If you're being a therapist, just turn them inwards towards their experience. You don't need to understand a thing.

(Kurtz 1985: iii)

Having in the last chapter established some theoretical orientations – worked out where north, south, east and west are, so to speak – in this chapter we begin to develop a map of the complex practice of body psychotherapy. (The epigraph above is to remind us not to get too hung up on complexity.) As with every psychotherapy, theory and practice operate in a dialectical relationship, each informing and changing the other. The chapter begins with a schema for relating the various theories of body psychotherapy to each other. Then we look at several concepts and terms which are central to the field, but either not used in other forms of psychotherapy, or used there in different ways. Finally, we survey the skills and techniques which are unique to body psychotherapy clinical practice.

Three models for body psychotherapy

Without drastically oversimplifying a fairly complex situation, we can identify three core models presently at work in body psychotherapy. In practice these are often not clearly described or distinguished, and are often used in combination or one after the other, despite some very real intellectual contradictions between them. These three models can be called the *Adjustment* model, the *Trauma/Discharge* model and the *Process* model. They do not operate solely in body psychotherapy, but can also be found in a number of verbal modalities. Each of the models, though, as we shall see, has a particular importance and relevance for body psychotherapy.

Unfortunately we cannot simply create lists of which schools of body therapy use which model. The models cut across the boundaries between schools – in fact, more often than not all three can be discovered in any given approach, though in varying proportions and with varying emphases. However, I think that understanding the three models still gives us a very useful tool for grasping and analysing the different schools of body psychotherapy, their similarities and differences.

The Adjustment model

The Adjustment model is the most controversial from a psychotherapeutic point of view. In the opinion of many body psychotherapists it should be banished to the realm of bodywork proper. It understands therapy as essentially a corrective treatment, which realigns the body – physically, energetically or both – and thus indirectly brings the mind back into a healthy and desirable condition. This view is clearly expressed, for example, in a passage from Lowen's classic work *Bioenergetics*:

> A person's emotional life depends on the motility of his body, which in turn is a function of the flow of excitation throughout it. Disturbances of this flow occur as blocks . . . Generally one can infer a block from seeing an area of deadness and sensing or palpating the muscular contraction that maintains it.
>
> (Lowen 1976a: 53)

Hence, by removing these blocks and increasing the flow of energy, one restores the patient to their healthy 'first nature' as opposed to the 'second nature' of neurosis (Lowen 1976a: 107).

This model – which Lowen inherits from one side of Reich's thinking – has several major limitations. First, it can be used in a way which crudely privileges the somatic over the psychological, assuming that it is always more effective to work from the body to the mind. Second, it has little immediate room for an appreciation of the complex protective and expressive functions of bodily 'disfunctions', the ways in which states of high or low tension can be the best available containers for a threatened sense of self. This understanding has been perhaps the major contribution of the 'second wave' of body psychotherapy. Nor does this model have much room for psychological phenomena like ambivalence, which are hard to translate into bodily terms. And third, of course, it assumes the practitioner's privileged understanding of what is best for the client, and her right to apply this understanding – literally 'manipulating' the client on a bodily level.

The Adjustment model is operating every time we use words like 'healthy', 'normal' or 'proper'. However hard we may try to move away from this view, it is deeply embedded in the traditions of body therapy and not so easy to dispose of. For example, in David Boadella's well-received speech to the First Congress of the World Council of Psychotherapy, one finds this:

> As motility is freed, one of the key physiological anchorings of character is loosened, with the result that outer movement expression becomes deeply connected to inner states of feeling; instead of flaccid or spastic states of armouring, the client connects with the gracefulness of movement.
>
> (Boadella 1997a: 33)

This is directly Reichian in tone and content and – as the case vignette to which Boadella moves on clearly shows – it is combined in Boadella's practice with both of the other two models I identify. However, it is worth insisting that this very familiar style of thinking about and looking at clients clearly privileges some particular concept of health and normality. Certainly in less skilled hands than Boadella's, such a style of thinking can set up a potentially stultifying transference/countertransference clash, where the therapist struggles to impose 'cure' (here, 'gracefulness of movement') on a client whose unconscious is deeply invested in their so-called 'disfunction'. I shall return to this issue in Chapter 5.

One might take it then that the Adjustment model is an outmoded positivist relic in the postmodern world, and that the only question is how best to do away with it. However this is not the view I want to put forward. I believe we have to recognize and take seriously the stubborn persistence in psychotherapy as a whole – not just in body psychotherapy by any means – of the idea of 'cure'. Cure is an easy concept to criticize, but it will not go away. In specifically body-psychotherapeutic terms, we cannot easily evade the body's wish for healing – which encompasses both the client's body wishing to be healed and the therapist's body wishing to facilitate healing. There are many crucial moments in psychotherapy of any kind where a stance on the therapist's part of offering cure would be disastrous to the work. However, this does not imply that cure itself is not a valid objective – the objective, in fact, which a *goal* of cure would put in jeopardy.

In reality, I suggest, every psychotherapist comes to the therapeutic encounter with their own strong notions of what constitutes health and good functioning. These views are not wholly susceptible to rational critique, since they constitute our categories of perception. This is particularly so for body psychotherapists, who are trained to identify somatic indicators of personality themes and issues. How are we to prevent ourselves from experiencing some bodies, say, as vital, upright and lithe, and other bodies as constricted, exhausted and collapsed? The most useful thing we can do, perhaps, is to cultivate a critical *awareness* of our own judgement, which allows us steadily to extend our acceptance of the different styles of embodiment which we encounter.

These considerations suggest that what needs scrutinizing is not so much the concept of adjustment itself, as the nature of the adjustment which we seek to facilitate. There are in fact at least two versions of Adjustment model in play in the field of body psychotherapy (and quite possibly for psychotherapy in general): one modelled on orthodox medical approaches, to which all the above strictures apply; the other deriving from or parallel to the approach of complementary healing, understanding adjustment as a matter of rebalancing, awakening and empowering the bodymind's own capacity to heal. Such an approach is necessarily respectful of the individual's self-understanding and goals, and seems to me consistent with the framework of psychotherapy.

The Trauma/Discharge model

The second model is the powerful theory of traumatic shock and reparative emotional discharge first formulated in modern terms by Freud and Breuer, who identified the origins of hysteria as 'psychical traumas which have not been disposed of by abreaction' (Freud and Breuer 1893–5: 66), and specifically related this to bodily symptoms and experiences: 'We must presume . . . that the psychical trauma – or more precisely the memory of the trauma – acts like a foreign body which long after its entry must continue to be regarded as an agent that is still at work' (1893–5: 56). This continues to be a central model for many body psychotherapists.

In his writings Freud repeatedly describes a core experience of attack, an external trauma which leads to defensive freezing (Freud 1909, 1920; Freud and Breuer 1893–5). Freud characterizes this as a 'foreign body', like a splinter or a parasite, which enters and attacks the child's bodymind so that their psychic structure has to adapt and shape itself around it. This adaptation, it seems, leads to the experience of *one's own bodily excitation* as a further attack, a second 'foreign body' which threatens the artificial defensive stasis precipitated by the original trauma, and which has to be dealt with by desperate measures (Freud 1926; Totton 2002a). Hence Freud even argues that strong emotions are 'universal, typical and innate hysterical attacks' (Freud 1926: 290) which take over the body in the same way as external trauma and undermine the bodymind's defensive stasis.

Although Reich does not explicitly use this concept of the 'foreign body', it is behind his whole conceptualization of repression, aggression and resistance. For Reich, our deepest resistance is against surrender and spontaneity – a freezing in the interests of survival in the face of external trauma. This theory is strongly supported by the evidence from neuroscience which we looked at in Chapter 2. Traumatic experience leads us to experience *our own body* as 'foreign'. If it seems vital to suppress feeling and emotional expression, then this can only be achieved by alienating ourselves from our own bodies, and 'senselessly defend[ing ourselves] against the cherished capacity for pleasure' (Reich [1942] 1983: 336).

Many versions of the trauma model in body psychotherapy are not as rich and subtle as this, however. They may amount only to the broad belief that bad experiences can get stuck in the body and need to be released in order for the bodymind to flourish. Such theories can be both oversimplified and over-optimistic: 'Pain is at the core of mental and physical illness – pain that comes from trauma and unmet needs . . . Early traumas leave a permanent imprint in the system . . . It is possible to relive these imprinted memories and resolve neurosis and physical disease' (Janov 1992: xxiii).

If the ruling metaphor of the Adjustment model is straightening a crooked limb, that of the Trauma/Discharge model is expelling a splinter which has created painful swelling and inflammation around itself. We should note that usually the body itself expels the splinter. Generally, the Trauma/Discharge model, like the 'complementary' Adjustment model described above, suggests that the practitioner's role is to support and encourage a natural healing. The Discharge part of the model argues that this healing occurs through emotional abreaction, the release and full conscious expression of the old emotions 'held' or 'locked' into rigid musculature.

How is this best to be done? Originally body psychotherapy tended simply to encourage intense emotional discharge as an absolute good, and this approach is still found. However, there is widespread understanding that a strong therapeutic relationship is an essential container for this process; and that for certain personality structures explosive discharge can be counter-productive and indeed damaging (Boadella 1987: 124). Currently there is a strong movement in body psychotherapy towards a more gentle and gradual approach to working with trauma, which avoids 'retraumatizing' the client, and focuses on supporting their strength and competence, on *managing* the traumatic memory rather than reliving it. But the basic model is still the same: that 'post-traumatic symptoms are, fundamentally, incomplete physiological responses suspended in fear', which 'will not go away until the responses are discharged and completed' (Levine 1997: 34; cf. Rothschild 2000, who shifts the emphasis even further from 'discharge' to 'completion').

Modern trauma theory is an excellent tool for approaching specific psychological wounds in given individuals – the whole area currently conceptualized as post traumatic stress disorder. Again, though, I would identify several limitations to this approach (the concept of PTSD itself is usefully critiqued in Bracken and Petty 1998 and in Leys 2000). First, as generally employed the Trauma/Discharge model does not fully incorporate transference and countertransference issues; in other words, it does not discuss the therapeutic contact itself as potentially a replication of trauma, which can be either creative or destructive, but in fact specifically tends to assume the therapist's position as friend and ally. (There are important exceptions to this, notably Rothschild 2000 and indeed Reich himself.)

As an extension of this, the model (especially in its more contemporary forms) often focuses on specifically and grossly traumatic events and not sufficiently on the universal, sub-critical trauma of socialization – the issues described in psychoanalysis under the rubric of the Oedipus complex (Laplanche and Pontalis 1988: 282–7). Third, and perhaps most importantly, the model may not address the profound questions about fantasy and external reality which trauma work raises, tending to assume a simple one-to-one relationship between what the client experiences in their bodymind and what has historically occurred. Anyone who works with birthing experiences, for instance, knows that clients can have deep experiences of birth, both positive and negative, which are very different from the birth process they actually underwent. The more sophisticated contemporary trauma therapists certainly acknowledge that 'memories' are not always factual; but they offer few tools for working with the non-factual element.

The Process model

Lastly, the Process model takes even further the idea of supporting a natural healing process. In fact in its pure form it drops the idea of 'healing' entirely, along with the idea of anything being wrong:

> If you want to help someone . . . turn the person inward towards experience. Don't turn them inward for explanations. Don't ask then why they feel that way – you're wrecking the process right there. You are taking the ship ashore. Don't ask for explanations. You don't need them. You don't need anything. It's not your problem. If you're being a therapist, just turn them inwards towards their experience. You don't need to understand a thing.
>
> (Kurtz 1985: ii-iii)

Working with the Process model, a therapist will allow the client's bodymind to guide the therapeutic journey, to act rather than be acted on, and to generate imagery and motifs freely and playfully. Hence the ruling metaphor here, rather than straightening a limb or expelling a splinter, is more like an improvised dance where the therapist follows the client:

> We try and follow the 'loose end of the string', unwinding the easiest thing that presents itself. We don't break through resistances

but instead follow the 'flow of the current', allowing an opening from the inside out, inviting the client to travel a little further than they think they can do on their own.

(Biosynthesis website, see Appendix)

At least while therapy is actually taking place, one is encouraged to let go of theory, and in particular let go of any concept of fixed states or entities. 'Our bodies are us as process, not as a thing. Structure is slowed-down process' (Keleman 1975: 66).

A great strength of the Process approach is that to a considerable degree it avoids the privileging of the therapist's version of reality, health and normality which I discussed above. All three are determined not by pre-existing theory, but by *what happens*, on the strong assumption that trauma and maladjustment will tend to self-repair given the slightest opportunity, and that the most apparently eccentric and bizarre behaviour can be part of this process. There is a close parallel with the concept of 'unwinding' in cranio-sacral therapy: 'inherent corrective physiological motion that can be induced from the nervous system' (Cohen 1995: 82).

Along with this strength go corresponding weaknesses. There is an uneasy relationship in most forms of process-centred body psychotherapy with *state*-based concepts like 'character', 'neurosis', etc. For example, Fritz Perls, who was strongly influenced by Reich, recognizes that 'the formation of character' allows the individual to 'act only with a limited, fixed set of responses' (Perls 1955: 4). He classifies types of such limited responses as five different interruptions of the 'cycle of creativity'. But Perls also insists that instead of trying to identify and treat 'the "real" underlying character that the therapist guesses at . . . we need only help the patient develop his creative identity' (Perls et al. [1951] 1973: 508–9). This reflects a general fear in process-oriented therapies of getting captured by the heavy gravitational field of state thinking, and losing one's capacity to fly freely.

But states are what we mostly inhabit; and state and process are inseparable and complementary concepts, each making sense of and delineating the other (Totton and Jacobs 2001: 111ff). A totally stable organism would be dead – metabolism implies change; but an organism which was all change would have no identity. Just as a cell needs a surrounding membrane to define it, human beings need 'edges' (Mindell 1985b) – psychological boundaries which resist change – in order to delineate where they are; in order to exist at all. One can think of these edges as our grip on embodiment. While it may be helpful to relax any particular edge, we cannot do without edges altogether.

More subtly, the laissez-faire ideology of process-centred approaches can license an informal, invisible domination by the therapist's views and predilections. Since the therapist's feelings and reactions are all 'part of the field', they can be brought in without restraint – and, as in all therapy, the practitioner is usually more relaxed and familiar with what is going on, giving them the potential to set the terms of the engagement. Process work often tends to be highly active and at times may insufficiently support the tendency to stay still – either stuck, which is often necessary and useful, or just 'being' rather than 'doing'.

Combining the three

The Hakomi Method, a modern form of body-oriented psychotherapy, is a good example of how the three models I am describing can coexist and interact. The dominant and explicit framework is the Process model, as shown by the quotation in the previous section. However, this exists alongside a strong and systematic Trauma model – a system of 'sensitivity barriers' which respond to deficits or traumas in the childhood environment and give rise to character structure. There is also an implicit assumption of the Adjustment model, as Kurt indicates:

> For example, the ability of the masochist to bear up under difficult conditions has left the same person with a slowness and seriousness that interferes with . . . the capacity to feel any *normal* sense of joy and lightness . . . the overdeveloped strengths of patience and bearing up lead to *malfunctions* in responsibility and the capacity to take action.
>
> (Kurtz 1985: 18/1–18/2; my italics)

This sort of entwining of the three models is the norm rather than the exception in contemporary body psychotherapy. It is also to be seen in the work of Wilhelm Reich, whom most body psychotherapists regard as the founder of the discipline. Reich frequently talks in terms of adjustment and correction, a 'concentrated attack' upon muscular and psychological rigidities (Reich [1942] 1983: 269); but he also draws very deeply on the Trauma/Discharge model. Reich seldom uses the actual term 'trauma', but the theory of psychic/somatic defence as a means of 'holding' old pain is central to his thinking, as appears in the same passage from which I have just quoted: 'Affects had broken through somatically after the patient had relinquished his attitude of psychic defense', embodied in a stiff neck ([1942] 1983: 269).

For Reich, undischarged feeling is literally *held* in muscular tension, of which psychological tension is the functional equivalent. As well as his investment in both the Adjustment and the Trauma/Discharge models, however, Reich also struggles towards what we can retrospectively see to be a process-centred view of body psychotherapy, encouraging clients to 'give in to every impulse' (Reich [1942] 1983: 311), and supporting these impulses without knowing in advance where they were leading (see Totton 1998: 107–12 for a detailed analysis along these lines of one of Reich's case histories).

As I have already indicated, although these three models often coexist in practice, as they did for Reich, there are important ways in which they conflict with each other. For example, if we work in terms of Adjustment, from the Process point of view we are interrupting the free unfolding of the client's material and imposing our own agenda. We may therefore also be retraumatizing the client, in terms of the Trauma/ Discharge model, by repeating the sort of interference which they experienced as children. If using a Process viewpoint, on the other hand, both the Adjustment and the Trauma/Discharge models argue that we may be skating over deep problems and colluding with the client by staying where they find it relatively easy to go. A Trauma/Discharge approach, in turn, can be seen from a Process point of view as backward looking and static, and from an Adjustment point of view as failing to restore healthy functioning.

But the existence of these clashes needs to be reconciled with the experiential fact that many or most body psychotherapists find they can in practice, at least to some extent (and not always consciously), make creative use of all three models, varying between them as different qualities of material emerge. The empirical usefulness of all three models suggests that there may be grounds for a new synthesis, for what one might call a General Theory of Body Psychotherapy, within which the three models will fall into place as three facets of a whole. I have more to say about this in Chapter 6.

Central concepts of body psychotherapy

At this point I want to pull together some ideas and theories that are central to body psychotherapy, and to explain what they mean and how they are used. Some of these are used in other forms of therapy, but in significantly different ways. Many are unique to the body psychotherapy tradition and many of them are referred to and discussed in various ways elsewhere in the book, but the most systematic account will be in the following section.

Bodymind, bodymindspirit

Bodymind is perhaps the most central of all body psychotherapy concepts, and I have already given a detailed account in Chapter 2. The bodymind concept treats each human being as essentially a unity, existing simultaneously and entirely in both the realm of embodiment and the realm of conceptualization. Many body therapists would also add the third realm of 'spirit' (see Chapter 6). From a practical point of view, this means that an individual can be approached and accessed equally from any of these viewpoints, as body, mind and/or spirit; the only question is which of these will be most useful at a given moment and in a given situation.

Embodiment

Another key concept which has already been used several times, 'embodiment' refers to the state of being united bodymind. It is often used to name the state of *experiencing* this unity. Conger (1994: 195) describes embodiment simply but resonantly as 'being at home in your body' – as opposed to being alienated from it, experiencing oneself as essentially a mind impeded or attacked by 'its' body. Hence the project of body psychotherapy is, in a sense, for the therapist to use her own embodiment, her own 'at-homeness', as a tool to help the client come into a similar state.

Functional identity

Our embodied status as united bodymind is the major example of Reich's theory of 'orgonomic functionalism', asserting what he calls the 'functional identity' of psychological and physiological processes: 'It would be wrong to speak of the "transfer" of physiological concepts to the psychic sphere, for what we have in mind is not an analogy but a real identity: the unity of psychic and somatic function' (Reich [1945] 1972: 340). This perception of course underlies the concept of bodymind; it also has specific applications to a number of other body psychotherapy concepts, as we shall see below.

Feeling

Body psychotherapists employ a bodymind understanding of emotion as simultaneously a psychological and a physiological event – an important example of functional identity. Many would conceptualize feeling *energetically* (see below). As Reich described his own theoretical development, 'the "emotions", more and more, came to mean manifestations of a tangible bio-energy, of the organismic orgone energy' (Reich [1945] 1972: xi). Emotion is 'e-motion', an outward movement: for body psychotherapists, it is part of the intrinsic nature of feelings to express themselves somatically and actively, and anything which interrupts this expression, while it may be unavoidable and even temporarily useful, is also inherently problematic.

Energy

Many or most forms of body psychotherapy make use of the term 'energy', but they mean several different things by it. Originally Freud called our sexual drive 'libido'. He understood this to be the central motivation of human existence and developed the concept into something more like life energy. Reich preserved a very literal, bodily sense of libido. He explored human bio-electricity and eventually believed himself to have discovered a concrete, literal life energy pervading the universe which he called orgone. Reich believed that orgone determined not only the state of the human body, but also weather phenomena and even the formation of galaxies: 'The same energy that guides the movements of animals and the growth of all living substances indeed also guides the stars' (Reich [1950] 1972: 94). Later Reichians and other body psychotherapists have several different readings of this concept. Radix, which in many ways stays closest to Reich's views, substituted for the physical-science concept of orgone the vision of a 'substratum from which energy and feeling are created and which forms the connecting link between the two. . . . something more fundamental than physical energy or force, something that is the simultaneous root of subjective experience and of bodily expression and movement' (Kelley 1974: vii).

Moving in the opposite direction, Alexander Lowen, founder of Bioenergetics, writes as if bioenergy – a term which he prefers to orgone – is much the same thing as straightforward metabolic energy (e.g. 1976a: 45–6).

Following on from Lowen, recent body psychotherapists tend to speak of 'energy' in a much looser and vaguer way. At the same time, however, the concept is often actually quite central to their practice. Therapists decide how to approach a client by their assessment of the state of the client's 'energy', and the perceived movement and variation in body 'energy' gives them crucial feedback on the effect of their interventions. For example, the Chiron Centre says of its work:

> Even when a session might look to an observer similar to any other form of psychotherapy – two people sitting together talking – a Chiron therapist would be using their perception of the client's energetic presence to gain a sense of all levels of the client's communication. The client would experience this mainly as a sense of being really listened to, and fully responded to. In using the word 'energetic' we are referring to the body/mind as a dynamic system, so that any look, gesture, phrase, etc. contains the essence (the energy) of an individual's life story.
>
> (Chiron website, see Appendix)

Most body psychotherapists would probably feel they understand this. Most other people, however, would be baffled – especially a physical scientist, who would conclude that the word 'energy' is being used here in a very unusual sense. And even body psychotherapists might find it very difficult to justify this sort of language. How, exactly, is the 'essence' of someone's life story a sort of 'energy'? How metaphorical or how literal is one being in talking like this? Often this sort of use of the word 'energy' refers to what we might call emotional tone – what Daniel Stern (1985) calls 'vitality affect' (see Chapter 2 and below). Sometimes there is an appeal to a specific energy model like those outlined below under the heading 'Subtle Body'.

There is a considerable body of research evidence now available which supports the idea of actual, physical body energy phenomena which can be communicated between one body and another, and which can be used to facilitate change in another body. The best account I know of this material is given by James Oschman (2000), who offers a series of complementary explanatory models for the experience of body energy, including electromagnetism, tensegrity theory, and the properties of the perineural system. The most fundamental model seems to be 'entrain-ment': the idea that energetic patterns existing in one organism will inherently tend to resonate with and be copied by another nearby organism. All this is still work in progress, but eventually may well offer a firm basis for energy formulations in body psychotherapy.

A number of bodyworkers would regard these details as irrelevant, but would perhaps agree with Richard Strozzi Heckler's formulation:

> Our energy is our aliveness. It is the stuff that creates the continuity of our life. We wake up with it, we go to bed with it, it is present in our waking and sleeping dreams. . . . It is the ground from which our living emerges. . . . In a way energy is nothing special, but it is the glue that binds everything together and connects us to our essential self.
>
> (Heckler 1984: 58–9)

Subtle body

One way to organize ideas about energy is through the traditional con-cept of the 'subtle body': a semi-material, semi-spiritual field which per-meates our physical being, and which can become blocked and distorted in parallel ways to our physical being (Cameron 2002). Hence, one can intervene on the subtle level just as one can on the bodily, the emo-tional or the intellectual level. Rose Cameron offers a number of terms for describing the vicissitudes of the energetic body field, including 'expansion', 'diffusion', 'contraction', 'clenching' and 'disembodying'. She argues that, energetically as physically, altering the state of the subtle body is a means of self-defence: 'however, like any other self-defence mechanism, it may become habitual and inappropriate, a problem rather than a solution' (Cameron 2002: 157).

There are a number of traditional 'maps' of the subtle body, many of them deriving from eastern spiritual and healing traditions, and body psychotherapists are often familiar with one or more of these; for example, Japanese and Chinese *chi* theory, the Indian system of *prana* and *nadis* which includes the well-known *chakras* or energy centres, and the various models of the 'aura' or energy field around the body. None of these models are interchangeable, nor can they be simply equated with Reich's orgone theory. The different energies have distinct and specific qualities. One cannot do acupuncture with orgone, or Reichian therapy with *prana*.

Flow, streaming, excitation, release

From the use of 'energy' as a central concept, whether metaphorically or literally, a whole series of other related terms follow for describing what that energy does or appears to do. This current group refers to the behaviour of energy which is not stuck or blocked, but able to move freely within the system of the human body. Energy can be seen and felt to flow, either outwards from the centre towards the periphery, or length-ways through the body – it was for this that Reich coined the name 'streaming' (Raknes 1971: 23–4). Lowen describes these phenomena as follows:

> Flow denotes a movement within the organism best exemplified by the flow of blood. . . . Energetically speaking, the whole body can be viewed as a single cell with the skin as its membrane. Within this cell excitation can spread in all directions or flow in specific directions depending on the nature of our response to a stimulus. . . . One can experience the flow of excitation as a feeling or sensation which often defies anatomical boundaries.
>
> (Lowen 1976a: 51–2)

Reich, however, insists that the 'vegetative currents' experienced in the body are not just the flow of blood and other fluids, but a specific 'bio-electricity' which is ultimately a form of orgone (Reich [1942] 1983: 272ff). Recent body psychotherapists usually take a more experiential attitude towards such issues.

Pulsation, contraction

For the Reichian tradition of body psychotherapy, the most basic function of embodied energy is pulsation: a rhythmic movement of spreading out and drawing in between centre and periphery. This can express itself in many forms, including breath, heartbeat, craniosacral rhythm, orgasm, and some forms of emotional expression: 'If you watch someone cry in pain or joy, you see that the whole person is convulsing rhythmically. It's interesting, because crying, unlike other forms of expression, almost always brings about the basic involuntary, pulsatory movements' (Keleman 1975: 20).

The most elaborate account of pulsation is found in Radix work, which centres its approach on restoring and supporting the free pulsation of the system, following Reich's dictum that 'if this biological state of pulsation is disturbed in one direction or in the other direction, that is if either the function of expansion or of the contraction predominates ... then a disturbance of the biological equilibrium in general is inevitable' (Reich [1942] 1983: 265). Radix divides pulsation into the *instroke* – the gathering of energy towards the core – and the *outstroke* – release of energy to the periphery and out into the world.

Recently Radix therapists have begun to focus on the positive importance of the instroke, distinguishing it from *counterpulsation* or actual contraction of the system: 'counterpulsation is armor in action' (Davis 1999a: 71). Contraction is the more common bodywork term and is seen as the fundamental factor limiting human pleasure and creativity:

When I speak of muscular contraction limiting the flow of energy, I am speaking of a deep, pervasive process. That is, I see every part of the body, including the organ systems, as functioning on the same principle of impulse formation, containment, transformation and expression of substances. Strong muscular contractions distort the bone structure development, tissue development, and even the chemical functioning of the body.

(Keleman 1976: 195–6)

One specific effect of contraction is that it interferes with free pulsation (Keleman 1976: 197–8).

Reichian theory uses the concept of pulsation to knit together phenomena from several different levels of experience, on the basis of functional identity:

On the highest psychic level, biological expansion is experienced as pleasure; contraction is experienced as unpleasure. In the realm of instinctual phenomena, expansion functions as sexual excitation, contraction functions as anxiety. On a deeper physiological level, expansion corresponds to parasympathetic functioning, and contraction to sympathetic functioning.

(Reich [1942] 1983: 289)

Charge/discharge

A closely linked concept in the Reichian tradition is the rhythmic cycle of energetic charge and discharge in the body. To function effectively, we need to charge ourselves up, for example, through breathing. Equally, we need to find adequate means of discharge and relaxation. For Reich, full discharge happens only through orgasm. Later neo- and post-Reichians have introduced much more complex and subtle ideas of charge and discharge.

Centre, centring, core

The idea of a centre or core is both metaphorical and literal, referring equally to a centre of the *self* and a centre of the *body*. 'Core space is the area in the body where there is unimpeded pulsation, i.e., where the system is unarmored' (Glenn and Muller-Schwefe 1999: 333). It is from this core space that energy expands outward into the rest of the body. This centre is generally understood to be in the viscera and the nerve plexi of the guts. Since it is the least armoured part of the system, contact with it is essential for well-being: 'Center is a basic bodily presence, and it is on this presence that the other bodily states are built. It is a bodily and energetic base camp' (Heckler 1984: 79). For Conger, a person's 'core signature' is their 'essential nature' which 'does not need fixing' (Conger 1994: 46). According to David Boadella:

> The therapeutic work of *centring* is concerned with re-establishing a functioning rhythm in the flow of metabolic energy and the balance between the two halves of the vegetative [autonomic] nervous system. In practice this means help towards recovering emotional balance and harmonious breathing.
>
> (Boadella 1987: 14)

From the Radix perspective and that of many others:

> Centering is . . . an absolute necessity in order to make contact with the individual, especially at the beginning of the work. It is an inward movement, first of all away from all demands, responsibilities and needs of the outer world. It is a concentration process, a focusing towards the inner world, the inner self.
>
> (Davis 1999b: 119)

Heckler emphasizes that we need to directly *experience* centring, rather than just subscribing intellectually:

The *idea* of center usually manifests itself as aloofness, detachment, rigidity, or some form of narcissism. From this idea, an attitude is shaped within the musculature, and soon we see a person who is thinking the idea of center but not experiencing it.

(Heckler 1984: 80)

Grounding

Equally as important as centring, and with a parallel functional identity of somatic and psychological meanings, is grounding. On one level this refers to a relaxed, responsive state of the leg musculature and a corresponding postural aliveness – only attainable if we have worked through traumatic aspects of the infant experience of standing unsupported. On another level, 'by channeling our energetic and bodily experience through our legs and into the earth, we become grounded in the living reality of our situation' (Heckler 1984: 86); so that 'not to know how one stands is equivalent to not knowing where one stands or to have no standing as a person' (Lowen 1976b: 185–6). Hence grounding can become a symbol of the whole state of embodiment:

To me, grounding means being anchored in our physical–psychic growth processes; expanding, contracting (contact, withdrawal), charging, discharging. Grounding means being rooted in and partaking of the essence of the human animal function. . . . Separation from the biological ground results in anguish and despair.

(Keleman 1976: 192–3)

One aspect of grounding, then, is to ground our conscious identity in our unconscious and involuntary self: 'The therapeutic work of *grounding* is concerned with establishing a good relationship between the voluntary, semi-voluntary and involuntary modes of movement and with recreating a more appropriate muscle tone' (Boadella 1987: 15).

An important distinction can be made (see Brown n.d.; Southgate 1980) between *vertical* and *horizontal* grounding. While Lowen, who introduced the concept of grounding to body psychotherapy, focuses on the upright posture and the leg-foot-ground relationship, as a basis for active involvement with the world, Reich's previous work can be understood as facilitating the equally legitimate and crucial ability to ground horizontally, to lie back and accept and surrender to the support of the earth. At different moments and for different people, either or both of these can be the important challenge.

Skying

Em Edmondson and myself (Totton and Edmondson 1988) have pointed out the equally significant function of 'skying' – the capacity to be in contact with those cosmic, visionary energies which we access through the crown of our head, as well as with the earth energies we access through our feet or sacrum. Unless we are grounded, this cosmic contact will be profoundly destabilizing (Cameron 2002); but similarly, without the sky connection, grounding will tend to become *over*-grounding, a heavy, stodgy practicality. Like a tree, human beings function best with their roots in the ground and their branches reaching for the heavens.

Facing

David Boadella's Biosynthesis (see Chapter 4) works with the three functions of centring, grounding and facing: 'Facing . . . is about having adequate contact with internal and external reality. This includes all our 'channels of contact' . . . especially the eyes and voice' (Labworth and Wilson 2000: 16). Boadella (1987: 16) suggests that working with facing is about finding a balance between over-sensitivity and under-sensitivity. As well as the eyes and voice, he connects it with 'the integration of language and perception with feeling' (1987: 16). These ideas relate closely to some of the neuroscience material outlined in Chapter 2.

Orgasm reflex, orgastic potency, genitality

For Reich and his orthodox followers, the goal and measure of health is what he calls 'orgastic potency' – not just the mechanical capacity for climax, but the ability to let go of all defence and control and abandon oneself wholly to the body. On the one hand, full orgasm of this kind is profoundly good for us; on the other, 'the capacity for complete surrender is one and indivisible, whether in a sexual embrace or in a task or in work' (Raknes 1971: 166). Hence, if we cannot surrender sexually we cannot ever release ourselves fully. One way in which a Reichian therapist assesses his client's degree of orgastic potency is through the 'orgasm reflex' – a gentle, non-sexual release of neck and pelvis with each outbreath, accompanied by streamings. Someone who is orgastically potent is, according to Reich, a 'genital character' – realistic, flexible, loving and freedom seeking (Reich [1945] 1972: 176ff).

Reich's focus on orgasm has been the subject of more revision than any other aspect of his work. Many neo- and post-Reichians have followed Lowen in making 'the shift from orgastic potency to pleasure as the therapeutic goal' (Lowen 1976b: 189). In some cases this is undoubtedly due to a strategic or characterological unwillingness to focus on sexuality as much as Reich did. However, there are good reasons for arguing that Reich exaggerated the role of sexual orgasm in achieving human health and happiness (Totton 1998: 99–101).

Self-regulation

This is another concept that invokes the idea of functional identity. Self-regulation in the first instance is a bodily state of free pulsation, not inhibited by contraction. The Reichian belief is that a person who is somatically self-regulated will also be self-regulated on a psychological level – that is, autonomous, self-motivated and appropriate. Hence self-regulation is very similar to the Reichian concept of genitality:

> Morality functions as an obligation. It is incompatible with the natural gratification of instincts. Self-regulation follows the natural laws of pleasure and is not only compatible with natural instincts; it is, in fact, functionally identical with them. . . . Steadily alternating between tension and relaxation, it is consistent with all natural functions. . . .
> The person with a healthy, self-regulated structure does not adapt himself to the irrational part of the world; he insists on the fulfilment of his natural rights.
>
> (Reich [1942] 1983: 181–2)

This also works the other way around: from a Reichian perspective, a person who is able to live a self-regulated life, without invasion by other people's attitudes and beliefs, is likely to be able to sustain somatic self-regulation as well: 'The most important condition for enabling the child to keep its free biological pulsation is self-regulation and the opportunity for alive contact with other people who are themselves tolerably free from anxiety and inhibitions' (Raknes 1971: 171). However children's natural, autonomous rhythm of life is very generally interfered with by the distress patterns of the adults around them. Reich points out that 'free, self-regulated behavior fills people with enthusiasm but at the same time terrifies them' ([1942] 1983: 183) and, when terrified, people tend to become aggressive and controlling.

Body memory

An important and controversial tenet of body psychotherapy is that the body can hold *memories* which do not exist in the conscious mind, but which can be accessed through various kinds of bodywork. Hence David Boadella argues that 'we do not need to limit memory . . . to the brain'

(Boadella 1987: 28), and discusses body memories from conception onwards. Reich does not go back so far, but asserts that *'every muscular rigidity contains the history and meaning of its origin'* (Reich [1942] 1983: 300; original italics). He describes many situations where the breakthrough of muscular impulse in body therapy is accompanied by both feeling and memory of the early life situation which created the original muscular block. Jack Rosenberg calls this sort of experience 'reliving' rather than remembering, because 'unlike remembering . . . it is a profound body mind experience involving all the senses – sight, hearing, smell, taste, touch. Simply remembering doesn't reach most of our early experiences because we had them before we had language. We retain the feelings in our bodies' (Rosenberg and Rand 1985: 28).

As we have seen in Chapter 2, there is now considerable research support for these ideas, particularly but not only as regards traumatic experiences. Research also supports the idea that more general 'state-dependent' body memories – potentially healing as well as traumatic ones – can be accessed through posture, movement, breathing, etc.

Shock, trauma

We have looked already in this chapter at the Trauma/Discharge model of body psychotherapy. The concept of shock or trauma can be used in a very concrete, practical way. Here is a bodyworker's description of trauma conceived as a physical/energetic phenomenon:

> A physical or an emotional blow can implode energy and create an area of increased entropy in the system. The body may respond by making a cyst to contain this entropy. This walling-off introduces an inertial state into the tissue. So you end up with an inertial phenomenon which is super-charged. We can take another leap from this and suggest that it will take a huge amount of energy to maintain this inertia around this 'super-charge'. So the body's resources will be continually sapped.
>
> (Ukleja 1998: 5)

In some ways this is very clear, in other ways very vague. It is an entirely literal, operational interpretation of the concept which many body psychotherapists will identify with, encountering localized trauma in the body in the form of 'stuck' or 'blocked' energy and seeking to release it as a discharge of pain, movement, sound and emotion (and perhaps also as memory). A sufficiently large trauma will also be seen to manifest as an overall body state of stuckness, rigidity or collapse.

A different way to conceptualize the same phenomena is in terms of the 'startle reflex', a whole-body contraction which is a baby's natural response to situations of alarm or shock, and an effective self-regulating way of discharging that shock. Continuing traumatized patterns can be seen as the result of a chronically interrupted startle reflex, so that the body has been unable to return to a state of relaxation. Shaking, trembling and sighing are other ways in which the body seeks to shake off the effects of trauma (Levine 1997), and these all tend to emerge in body psychotherapy.

Birth, birthing

The primary, universal trauma of human life, according to a number of body psychotherapists, is birth: 'Birth is a formative drama which can potentiate some of our deepest personality patterns. . . . Any understanding of later character dynamics rests on this first engagement with the outside world' (Boadella 1987: 38). Many practitioners, as they work with their clients, are holding the image of birth somewhere in the back of their minds as a possible template for their client's experience. This template will be brought into the foreground if the client, for example, talks about feeling 'under pressure' or 'squeezed', mentions 'light at the end of the tunnel', or produces bodily symptoms like a pressure headache or emotional symptoms like premonitions of disaster. A range of different methods for 'birthing' or 'rebirthing' the client has been developed and some of these are discussed in Chapter 4 as 'primal therapies'. Some body therapists specialize in this area, and many others include it somewhere in their tool kit.

Armouring

Reich coined the term 'armouring' to describe systematic patterns of chronic muscular rigidity, which he likened to armour in that they are hard, tough, restrictive, and have a protective function (Reich [1942] 1983: 299ff). We develop armouring in response to situations of chronic trauma – generally the trauma of socialization rather than any more dramatic events – through habitually inhibiting our impulses of emotional expression. Holding back crying, anger, etc. sets up muscular armouring. For Reich, armouring begins with holding our breath so as not to feel and spreads out from there. Armouring both embodies repression and preserves the repressed impulse itself.

Muscular armouring is functionally identical with *character* armouring, the systematic patterns of chronic psychological rigidity that also act to protect us from internal and external danger. This was one of the ways in which Reich realized that body and mind are one: 'If the character armor could be expressed through the muscular armor, and vice versa, then the unity of psychic and somatic functioning had been grasped in principle' (Reich 1983: 271).

Character

In the Reichian tradition of body psychotherapy (Reich [1942] 1983; Totton and Jacobs 2001: 35ff), a person's character is the ensemble of their various armourings, the complex chord created by all the various notes of repression and inhibition sounded in their history. Character structure – what Richard Strozzi Heckler calls our 'conditioned tendency' – is the chronic enactment of traumatic crises. Character traits embody both the original desire of the child and its repression through fear of outside reaction. 'A person's character conserves and at the same time wards off the function of certain childhood situations' (Reich [1945] 1972: 305).

Since 'the psychic structure is at the same time a biophysiological structure' (Reich [1942] 1983: 300–1), then it follows that bodily structure will vary with psychic structure; and this indeed is Reich's theory of character – character is the *embodiment* of trauma and defence. Different character structures give rise to different body shapes and attitudes, so that a skilled person can 'read' the key themes and issues of someone's life from their inscription on the body (Dychtwald 1978; Kurtz and Prestera 1976; Lowen 1958; Reich [1945] 1972). It is not possible here to describe the variety of character systems within the Reichian tradition (see Totton and Jacobs 2001), but all versions are derived from a shared model in which frustrating object relations impact on infant development during specific activation phases.

Reichian character theory is both powerful and illuminating. It offers a model of individual difference which is historically, somatically and politically inflected (character positions originate through our experience of power relations, in the policing of our bodily functions). However, it has tended to be downplayed or even ignored in many recent versions of body psychotherapy. This seems to result from a humanistic unease about 'pigeonholing' people. Certainly character theory can be misused if it is adapted to a medicalized approach of diagnosis and treatment. But the theory itself is precisely a subtle account of *individuality in relationship*, and of the strategies and defences used to preserve individual freedom – and the price paid in doing so:

> In the course of our development we make certain choices, consciously and unconsciously, to ensure our physical, social and emotional survival. These kinds of choices create attitudes that, in turn, shape our experience of the world. . . . The choices that lead to the forming of attitudes involve some sort of compromise, so what

we do is sacrifice some part of ourselves in order to survive. . . . In a sense this self-wounding is an intelligent act in that it is necessary for survival; at the same time, it also becomes the core of our neurosis.

(Heckler 1984: 20)

One can actually go a good deal further in rehabilitating the concept of character and point out that embodiment necessarily has to take some *form*, and that any form implies limitation. From this perspective, character is simply the specific form which a person's creative impulse takes. However, this can become damagingly limited if their options and understanding are reduced to a single key for all life's locks. If 'a person's character is the functional sum total of all past experiences' (Reich [1942] 1983: 145), then it embodies all our joys and triumphs as well as all our suffering.

The theory of character and muscular armouring looks at the effects of traumatic interaction on the quality of voluntary control over particular muscles and muscle groups. For example, the anal sphincter is not under voluntary control in a human infant. Pressure from carers to be 'clean' before voluntary control is achieved can only be met by tensing the whole body area – a tension accompanied, no doubt, by fear and shame. Clearly the *quality* of control in the anal sphincter itself, once achieved, is going to be different as a result: this sort of gross tension will disturb the development of fine, precise voluntary control.

Since our voluntary musculature in general has a differential development rate – we spend several years gradually attaining control of our movements, and in each muscle group gross motor control also occurs before fine control – command of the voluntary musculature can in theory be mapped in detail onto developmental sequence, so that traumatic interactions will appear as a disturbance in specific body areas, and affect the final shape, movement and postural style of the adult body. This mapping has already been attempted (Bentzen and Bernhardt 1992).

Sensory-motor amnesia

Sensory-motor amnesia is a useful term coined by Thomas Hanna as a redescription of what Reich referred to as 'armouring':

Constant repetition of stressful stimuli will cause loss of conscious voluntary control of significant areas of the body's musculature . . . these areas of musculature can be neither voluntarily sensed nor controlled. The victim can attempt to relax his amnesic lumbar muscles voluntarily, for example, but he no longer has the ability to do so; both the sensing and movement of these muscles are beyond the reach of his voluntary control. The muscles remain rigid and immobile, as if they belonged to someone else.

(Hanna 1997: 349–50)

In other words, stress – including sustained trauma – can alienate us from our body awareness, in a way which cannot be reversed simply by will; a process which, as Reich points out, is functionally identical to Freud's discovery of psychological repression: 'Muscular rigidity, wherever it occurs, is not a "result", and "expression", or a "concomitant" of the mechanism of repression. In the final analysis . . . somatic rigidity represents the most essential part of the process of repression' (Reich [1942] 1983: 300).

A good deal of the activity of bodywork and body psychotherapy, from this perspective, can be seen as attempts to dissolve sensory-motor amnesia. Hanna refers to this as 'somatic learning':

> If one focuses one's awareness on an unconscious, forgotten area of the soma, one can begin to perceive a minimal sensation that is just sufficient to direct a minimal movement, and this in turn gives new sensory feedback of that area which, again, gives new clarity of movement, etc. . . . This back-and-forth motor procedure gradually 'wedges' the amnesic area back into the range of volitional control.
> (Hanna 1997: 350)

Body psychotherapy, as distinct from bodywork, contributes to this process an awareness of the psychological resistance to 'remembering' our body, a process which of course includes remembering the reasons for our amnesia.

Motor patterning

Motor patterning is one term and technique for contacting the body's impulse to movement, repressed and preserved through armouring: 'The biosynthesis therapist can pick up an arm or other body part and ask what it wants to do, i.e. discover its motor patterning' (Labworth and Wilson 2000: 17). Many body therapists work in this sort of way, but only recently has the approach been articulated – perhaps most eloquently in Biosynthesis:

> We are working in a dialectical way between verbal and non-verbal communication, seeking to find a bridge between inner ground and outer reality. The work is with specific patterns of movement intentionality . . . We would ask clients questions as we work with these 'motor fields' such as: 'What kind of gesture do you want to do as you tune into your arm?', or 'How does it feel to push me away?' These patterns are deeply connected to developmental neuromuscular sequences in prenatal life, during birth and in childhood.
> (Biosynthesis website, see Appendix)

Contact

> How strange it seems that, despite its power to heal and inspire, contact plays such a small part in our education and healing professions, to say nothing of our everyday life.
>
> (Heckler 1984: 118)

For body psychotherapists, contact is an essential prerequisite of the work and also a quality which the work strives continuously to deepen. Again, the term is a metaphor derived from bodily experience: it describes the state of being 'in touch', with oneself, with the world, or with another person. Contact is what makes the difference between touching one's lover or child and touching the person next to one on a commuter train. It is a condition of living relationship, which, as Gestalt therapy reminds us, depends on the ability to create a boundary between self and other: 'contact is the appreciation of differences' (Fritz Perls, quoted in Heckler 1984: 119).

Armouring and contraction create a state of contactlessness (Reich [1945] 1972: 308ff). The individual may wear a mask of vitality and sociality, but is fundamentally out of touch with their own somatic and emotional experience, and similarly out of touch with the world around them and with other people. By uninvasively offering the client embodied contact – which may or may not include physical contact – the body psychotherapist seeks to reawaken their ability to feel both self and other.

Presence

In order to offer contact, the therapist – or any person – needs to be fully present to their own being. This capacity flows from our ability to own and accept all aspects of our own experience, including feelings and impulses that may at first seem shameful or frightening:

> Contact can take almost any form as long as we bring an energetic presence to the form. Contact is how we are with somebody or something. Presence, which is our embodied awareness, is the mother of contact. Contact is the process of transmitting meaningful information . . . and it originates in our living presence.
>
> (Heckler 1984: 119)

Attention, awareness

Attention is the act of focusing awareness on some particular aspect of our experience. Bringing conscious awareness to our experience is the fundamental mechanism of change (Mindell 1985a). It is also, of course, very difficult! We defend against awareness of experience which is too painful; hence all the techniques of psychotherapy for recovering awareness. At the same time, though, awareness is constantly trying to happen: 'The processes which you perceive, your focus, channel changes, edges, problems and illnesses are organized in such a way as to make you aware as quickly as possible of how your secondary process conflicts with your primary one' (Mindell 1990: 123). Mindell uses 'primary process' to indicate the aspects of our experience with which we currently identify, and 'secondary process' for those aspects which we currently take to be 'other'.

Our somatic experience is a powerful field for developing awareness and attention: 'Our attention is similar to an organ or muscle in that it functions within the biological domain and can be cultivated, nurtured, and strengthened through bodily practices' (Heckler 1984: 60–1). Working with repressed experience on the bodily level allows for very precise focus, and can sidestep some forms of psychological avoidance. If we feel a pain in a particular muscle, for example, we can use various methods to bring our awareness to that exact spot – including breath, voice, tensing the muscle, putting pressure on it, etc. Once we actually become aware 'from the inside' of how we are holding on with the muscle, we automatically become able to relax it and the experience which we are holding back automatically enters our awareness.

Micro-movement

This is an increasingly important concept in the USA, especially in the 'somatics' network. It brings together several forms of contemporary bodywork – notably craniosacral therapy – with body psychotherapy, focusing on very slight, subtle and spontaneous impulses in the body which are completely outside conscious awareness.

'A micro-movement resembles a subatomic pulsation of light, the smallest visible bit of movement' (Conrad Da'oud 1997: 70). It generally takes the form of a fine tremor or vibration. By bringing our attention to micro-movements and relaxing into them, we bring that part of the body to life, so to speak, generating a richness of sensation and activity which can be transformative. The focus on micro-movement is part of a very general tendency in both body psychotherapy and bodywork towards minimalism and least-intervention approaches.

Unique skills of body psychotherapy

Body psychotherapists need all the generic skills that any psychotherapist should have: technical ones like accurate listening, the ability to track one's own feelings and fantasies, or channel identification, and more fundamental 'meta-skills' (Mindell 1995) like patience, kindness and courage. There are also certain additional skills which are specific to the context of body psychotherapy, or which perhaps take on a different form in that context.

Contact

We have already considered the concept of contact and its important role in this work. Body psychotherapists need specific skills in this area: the ability to recognize the presence or absence of contact, to track it as it waxes and wanes, to offer it in the form and channel most acceptable to the client, and in a way which is both firm and unthreatening. Sometimes contact will be offered through touch. Like a massage therapist, the body therapist needs to have developed a relaxed, warm, confident, reassuring and gentle touch. Hands which are cold and clammy, abrupt, tentative or invasive will not convey an invitation to contact.

This implies that the practitioner will need to understand and work through their own issues around touch. Something similar is true about contact in general – it is not just a technical skill, more a way of life. Richard Strozzi Heckler says:

> Establishing contact with ourselves naturally creates the foundation for purposeful contact with others and the environment. We must first learn how to be with ourselves before we can truly be with others. . . . When we are connected with ourself, our excitement automatically begins to flow outward, and we weave the fabric of our lives with the streamings and pulsations of those around us.
>
> (Heckler 1984: 122)

Intricate tactile sensitivity

Beyond the basic yet subtle issue of high quality touch, body psychotherapists frequently cultivate what Don Hanlon Johnson (2000) calls 'intricate tactile sensitivity' (ITS). As well as giving and receiving contact, they are also using touch to pick up complex information about the immediate and long-term state of their client's embodiment; and also to influence that state in subtle ways through the quality of their touch.

Johnson identifies three elements which define ITS. The first of these he terms '*discreteness*': the ability to discriminate different sorts of information received through touch, including micro-movements in the client's body, variations in temperature, tissue density and tissue tone, different pulsations, and different reactions to touch – variations of resistance, receptivity, etc.

The second element is *'pattern sensitivity'*: a non-verbal sensitivity to movements throughout large segments of the body, which can be contacted from touch at one point, so that the practitioner experiences their awareness 'reaching out' into the client's whole body and identifying patterns which are then given names like 'blocks', 'pulls', 'twists', 'shears', and so on.

The third element he calls *'sensitive contact'* between therapist and client, a unique level or flavour of contact which derives from this deep tactile connection. This is certainly something which many people who use ITS will recognize: a profound intimacy which grows out of the sense that one is touching the *inside* of a person's body, cupping their organs and swaying to the tides of their fluid systems.

Johnson is primarily discussing bodywork approaches such as Alexander Technique, Craniosacral Therapy and Continuum Movement, rather than body psychotherapists. Many body psychotherapists have actually trained in one or more of these modalities, or learnt similar skills as part of their body psychotherapy training; but even those who have not, if they use touch in their work, have generally developed intuitive ITS skills, although these may not be as consciously accessible or easily articulated. Some therapists conceptualize ITS information as referring to qualities of subtle energy rather than to physical phenomena. (Of course this may equally happen the other way round.)

Bonnie Bainbridge Cohen offers a helpful example of how the use of ITS may be conceptualized and experienced by the practitioner:

> All living organisms respond to touch and movement in a palpable way. Changing the quality of touch in subtle ways can elicit different and equally subtle responses. The awareness of these intricate and complex interactions involves the perceiving of delicate changes in breathing, the expanding and condensing of the membranes of the cells in the different layers of tissues, and the flow of fluid between the cells. These activities establish the pathways of the micromovements throughout the body that create the blueprint for the movements of our body through space.
>
> (Bainbridge Cohen 1997: 19)

Proprioception

Paralleling this deep connection with the client's body, body psychotherapists need an equally deep connection with their own embodied life. This follows from what I said earlier about contact: that we need to be in contact with ourselves in order to be in contact with others. Just as we are learning about the client's embodiment when we touch them, so (usually less consciously) they are learning about ours. This is the basis of the Alexander Technique, where teachers convey a particular postural quality to the client through embodying it as they touch them.

Hence, we need to know what we are embodying! As we work, a part of our attention needs to be tracking our posture, our breathing, our state of alertness, relaxation or tension, the coming and going of pains, itches and other stimuli. This not only enables us to model embodiment for our clients, instead of preaching something we aren't doing, but also connects us with a major source of information about what is happening in the room, how the client's presence is affecting us, what transactions are taking place between these two bodies in relationship:

> Our bodies are constantly sending and receiving information. In the therapy hour I watch not only the client's energy but also my own. I observe not only the client's breathing and constrictions, but I also attend to my own. . . . I feel what sensations emerge in my own body as the client works.
>
> (Conger 1994: 20)

Much as a psychodynamic therapist will track their own associations and fantasies as they sit with the client, a body psychotherapist – who may well be doing the same – will also track their body life. Focusing, an approach developed by Ernest Gendlin, is a powerful tool for connecting with and tracking one's embodied experience; and a number of body therapists use it for this purpose. I discuss Focusing in Chapter 4.

Body reading

Body psychotherapists tend to have highly developed skills of observing and interpreting the body (Kurtz and Prestera 1976). Many sets of categories are used for this, including Reich's original model of seven bodily segments (Reich 1972: 368ff; Totton and Edmondson 1988: Chapter 4), and distinctions between left/right, top/bottom, front/back, etc. (Dychtwald 1978; Smith 1985: 74–80). Depending on the therapist's specific orientation (so to speak), they may also consider the client's capacity to ground (Lowen 1976a), to centre or face (Boadella 1987), to sky (Totton and Edmondson 1988); whether their structure is over- or underbound, swollen, rigid, dense or collapsed (Keleman 1985); or where they appear to fit into a set of character structures (Totton and Jacobs 2001: 35ff).

They may also use much more intuitive and inexplicit ways of grasping the 'individual signature of the body' (Conger 1994: 45). For example, they may work with metaphor and imagery, perceive the client as a particular animal or plant, ask themselves 'what sort of child do I see in this adult?', and hold their own body in the posture of the client, to see what it feels like. Conger distinguishes three levels at which we can read the body: the 'initial signature', self-conscious presentation, showing either disguise or vulnerability; the 'shadow signature', the pattern of defences; and the 'core signature', the 'essential nature' which 'does not need fixing' (1994: 46).

Some body psychotherapists have an ability to 'read off' a client's history in some detail from looking at their body. This may work on an intuitive level – there is a considerable mystique around this talent – or be highly analytic, as with Lisbeth Marcher's Bodynamic system which looks at each muscle group's position on a scale of rigidity/flaccidity and relates this to a precise childhood sequence of muscle activation (Bentzen and Bernhardt 1992).

Vitality affect reading

As we have already seen, 'vitality affect' is Daniel Stern's (1985) term for dynamic emotional qualities expressed in a range of modalities including movement and voice. These qualities are central to the work of the body psychotherapist. One suspects that they manifest also in the sorts of information picked up through ITS. Body psychotherapists need to be able to perceive, discriminate, and have some sort of language to name vitality affects. By the very nature of vitality affects, this language is likely to be highly metaphorical:

> Others frequently ward off their repressed aggression by 'insinuating' – as one such patient once put it – themselves into the favour of any person capable of rousing their aggression. They become as 'slippery' as eels, evade every straightforward reaction, can never be held fast. Usually, this 'slipperiness' is also expressed in the intonation of their voice; they speak in a soft, modulated, cautious, and flattering way. In taking over anal interests for the purpose of warding off the aggressive impulses, the ego itself becomes 'greasy' and 'slimy' and conceives of itself in this way.
>
> (Reich [1945] 1972: 175)

Affect attunement

Body psychotherapists also need to be able to achieve affect *attunement*: to match and feed back to the client their pattern of vitality affect, as a way of both making contact and amplifying the client's patterns. Much of this work may be unconscious on both sides, but it is crucial, allowing the therapeutic relationship to mirror and perhaps to repair the infant's experience of developing social capacities through attunement which we explored in Chapter 2. This capacity for attunement is probably crucial for effective psychotherapy of any kind; but body psychotherapists have perhaps a greater ability to bring some of it to conscious awareness, and to play deliberately with matching and exaggerating vitality affects.

This comes out particularly clearly in dance movement therapy, where mirroring and non-verbally commenting on the client's movement patterns is a core technique:

> Mirroring, as emotional attunement, draws attention to an essential ingredient of the psychotherapeutic process. . . . In the end it is our ability . . . to recognise and mirror empathically the expressive reactions of our patients which is fundamental to the success of psychotherapy.
>
> (Chodorow 1991: 7; cf. Siegel 1984)

It is also found in other forms of body psychotherapy, and like so many other techniques was pioneered by Reich:

> I began to hold up a mirror to his behavior. When I opened the door to let him in, he would be standing there with a sullen, pain-distorted face, the epitome of a bundle of misery. I imitated his appearance. I began to speak to him in his childish language; I also lay on the floor and kicked and screamed the same way he did. At first he was astonished, but broke out in a spontaneous laugh one time, completely mature, completely unneurotic. . . . I continued these procedures until he himself began to analyze. Now we were able to continue.
>
> (Reich [1945] 1972: 244)

Many body therapists think in terms of *energetic* attunement, 'tuning in to' their client's patterns of body energy, as described in the previous section (e.g. Pierrakos 1987). It is a matter of opinion whether this is a separate skill, or a different conceptualization of affect attunement.

Bodywork

Several body psychotherapy approaches include in their range of techniques hands-on bodywork skills which one might describe as more interventionist than the ITS techniques mentioned above. The most well known of these are those Reichian schools which use deep pressure to force the release of muscle tension and break up restrictions in the connective tissues (Baker 1980; Painter 1984).

Another important technique is biodynamic massage (Boyesen 1980; Carroll 2002a), which uses a different set of techniques, some 'deep' and some 'gentle', towards the same goals (see Chapter 4). Bioenergetics and some other approaches use exercises and postures to raise energy levels and release blocks (Lowen 1976a, 1977); while dance movement therapy, of course, has its own highly developed forms of kinesthetically oriented bodywork.

As with the other skills described here, a great deal of training is needed in order to use bodywork effectively and appropriately. An essential component of that training is direct embodied experience of the work, which educates the intuition and motor-vestibular memory (see Chapter 2) as well as the conscious mind.

Breathwork

An integral aspect of bodywork for Reichians and many other body psychotherapists is work with the breath. Reich pointed out that the fundamental way in which we stop ourselves *feeling* is to stop ourselves *breathing*:

> Imagine that you have been frightened or that you anticipate great danger. You will involuntarily suck in your breath and hold it. . . . You will soon breathe out again, but the respiration will not be complete. It will be shallow. . . . It is by holding their breath that children are in the habit of fighting against continual and tormenting conditions of anxiety which they sense in the upper abdomen. They do the same thing when they sense pleasurable sensations in the abdomen or in the genitals, and are afraid of these sensations. . . . The way in which our children achieve this 'shutting-off feeling in the stomach', with the help of respiration and abdominal pressure, is typical; and universal. . . . In reduced respiration, less oxygen is introduced . . . With less energy in the organism, the vegetative excitations are less intense and, therefore, easier to control.
> (Reich [1942] 1983: 306–9)

Hence all forms of neo- and post-Reichian psychotherapy place great emphasis on restoring the client's capacity to breathe fully and freely. Some intervene directly and forcefully to 'break down' the muscular blocks against breathing, notably in the diaphragm. Others focus on supporting the sense of safety and relaxation so that the breath will naturally and gradually deepen. It is not a matter of willed, deliberate deep-breathing, but of surrender to our spontaneous breath: 'The experience of breathing provides the most continuous lived bodily form for the ego's fundamental experience of itself. . . . As one patient reported:

"When I feel my breathing fully, I feel as though I've come into the clear."' (Eigen 1993: 44–5).

Because free, full breathing involves surrender, it is deeply bound up with the therapeutic relationship. As with free association in psychoanalysis, the client can only allow themselves to open up this deeply if they trust their therapist equally deeply. Hence a focus on breathing brings up transference material and, because the experience is intimate and stirring for both participants, countertransference material. At the same time, and very importantly, better contact with the breath also *supports* our courage to relate:

> In breathing the insides of the body are continuously fed by the outside world, a continuous interpenetration of bodily depths and open expanses. This basic, sustaining interpenetration provides a bodily form for communion and relatedness in life. It helps support the current of hope and trust in personality since it is virtually in every moment in the process of giving one gratification.
>
> (Eigen 1993: 45)

Breathwork in body psychotherapy can induce a phenomenon known medically as 'hyperventilation': the breath becomes both intense and apparently unstoppable, accompanied by painful cramps in the hands, feet, face and other areas, and often by panic on the part of the breather. Physiologically speaking, this happens because the breather has over-emphasized their outbreath, blowing too much carbon dioxide out of the body and temporarily changing their blood and muscle chemistry.

Some forms of body psychotherapy – for example, Rebirthing and Holotropic Breathwork – deliberately induce this state. Others accept it as a fairly common effect of focus on the breath. (Even if one refrains from encouraging deeper breathing, but simply invites people to bring their awareness to their breath – as in Embodied-Relational Therapy, for example – hyperventilation still sometimes happens.) It is empirically certain that someone who is hyperventilating can be encouraged and supported to 'go through' the experience and find their way to a deep, grounded and balanced breath. The experience is usually profoundly rewarding and freeing for the person involved and often confers a degree of 'immunity' against hyperventilating in future. What helps a person go through hyperventilation is encouragement to make sound with their voice and to use the cramped muscles to squeeze, hit or kick out, together with reassurance that the process is natural and OK.

Hence, from an energetic point of view, it seems what is happening is that bodily blocks against expressing emotion, which have been amplified through deep breathing, are overcome and definitively released. What is happening physiologically is less clear. Hyperventilation is certainly a powerful, sometimes frightening, and occasionally dangerous tool, which no one, client or practitioner, should use without deliberate and informed choice. Some body psychotherapists are in fact opposed to its use (e.g. Boadella 1987: 80–3). Spontaneous hyperventilation can usually be mechanically dampened down by giving the person a paper bag to breathe into and out of, thus restoring carbon dioxide to the body.

Somatic countertransference

Countertransference, of course, refers to the emotional and fantasy reactions which the therapist has to the client, equivalently to the client's transference reactions to the therapist. Countertransference can be an enormously valuable tool for understanding the client's issues, as we are 'dreamt up' to portray various roles from their internal life. 'Dreaming up' is a technical term from Process Oriented Psychology, which neatly describes the way in which we often find ourselves embodying other people's internal figures.

Body psychotherapists need to understand these issues and be comfortable with their own reactions just as much as any other psychotherapist. They also need to be comfortable and familiar with a particular set of countertransference reactions which happen in and through their body:

> I very often get 'symptoms' when a patient begins a session or after some moments of work. These are usually bodily reactions of various kinds, such as headaches, stomach aches, heartaches, shortness of breath, sphincter tensions, fatigue, etc. They do not usually have a direct connection with what is being said, but whenever I reveal these reactions, I almost always discover that the patient is having, or had in the recent past, the same symptom or one related to it. Most of the time an underlying symbolic parallel is associated to the psychological content being discussed.
>
> (Spiegelman 1996: 114)

Similarly, Arnold Mindell says:

> Each of us knows what it is like to be dreamed up physically. How 'uptight' or nervous we feel in certain people's neighbourhood. How we get stomach cramps, headaches and other symptoms apparently in reaction to someone's behavior. These same reactions appear in therapists along with strong physical signals such as being exhausted by a [client], being turned on or off sexually . . . getting cramps, becoming nervous, suddenly becoming happy or sad, etc.
>
> (Mindell 1985: 48)

These phenomena are powerful enough to have been recognized by several practitioners who do not identify themselves as body psycho-therapists. The psychoanalyst Theodore Jacobs suggests:

> The analyst's own bodily responses as he listens to, or otherwise interacts with, the patient can assist him in his analytic work. By monitoring his own kinesic behavior as it occurs in response to his shifting psychological state, he may be able to put himself more finely in tune with his unconscious reactions. This increased self-awareness can then be used, either in the service of providing clues to the meaning of the patient's communications, or in facilitating the recognition of previously undetected attitudes and feelings in the analyst himself.
>
> (Jacobs 1973: 77)

Jacobs offers several case vignettes, including the example of a client who maintained an extended resistance to offering any meaningful material:

> Faced with what I considered so little interpretable material, I became increasingly silent, and as I did so, the patient's hostility grew. Then, one day, I observed the two of us: the patient as rigid as a coiled spring, his elbows protruding like iron pickets, and I, folded into myself, my arms wrapped across my chest, maintaining a grim and stubborn silence. . . . Out of sheer frustration I had locked horns with the patient, and my silence was, in great measure, a retaliation. Consciously, I told myself there was nothing to say, but, in fact, my body posture spoke for me: I was not going to say anything. The analysis had deteriorated into a struggle over who would control it, and it was rapidly becoming a stand-off.
>
> (Jacobs 1973: 89)

Several Jungian analysts have also identified somatic countertransference under one name or another (e.g. Jacoby 1986; Schwartz-Salant 1982). In particular, Andrew Samuels (1989: 150ff) distinguishes between 'reflexive' and 'embodied' countertransference, the latter being close to 'dreaming up':

> 'Embodied' is intended to suggest a physical, actual, material, sensual expression in the analyst of something in the patient's inner world, a drawing together and solidification of this, an incarnation by the analyst of a part of the patient's psyche and . . . a 'clothing' by the analyst of the patient's soul.
>
> (Samuels 1989: 151)

Whether we call it 'somatic' or 'embodied' countertransference, 'somatic resonance', 'somatic empathy', 'dreaming up', or something else, this capacity for embodied relationship – including all of the irrational and projective elements of relationship in general – is a tremendously important tool for body psychotherapy. It is also identified as important in Dance Movement Therapy (e.g. Chodorow 1991: 7; Siegel 1984: 120ff). It can be argued that the use of somatic countertransference, with no other specifically body-oriented tools, is in itself sufficient to qualify the work as body psychotherapy (Roz Carroll, personal communication).

CHAPTER 4

Varieties of body psychotherapy

The multitude of systems suggests an uninvented cosmology of health.

(Grossinger 1995, Vol. 2: 351)

Like a tropical jungle, the body psychotherapies at first present a confusing riot of forms, and any system imposed on them is to some extent an artificial aid to comprehension. Individual approaches change and grow over time, take on new influences and develop new understandings; Schools cross-fertilize with each other and bear new fruit. Richard Grossinger is right as well to point out that often at least: 'The real somaticists are not the ones who are most public with their work but those hidden away in nooks and crannies, improving on their own or as small clusters in collaborative training groups' (Grossinger 1995, Vol. 2: 198).

In other words, many excellent body psychotherapists – and this is true also of verbal therapists, though less so than formerly – are only notionally aligned with any particular existent 'method'. Primarily, they are doing what works for them, having long ago digested their original training into an often idiosyncratic personal approach. Grossinger also suggests: 'Nothing distinguishes popular bodywork of the 1980s and 1990s so much as its movement away from Reich's model of character armour and orgastic potency toward a multiple variety of circumstances of character resistance, armour, co-ordination, and intrinsic energy' (1995, Vol. 1: 422–3).

Although there is some truth in this, at least locally to California, it may itself already be a dated perception: interest in Reich's work has revived and deepened over the last decade. Certainly he is still by far the biggest star in the body psychotherapy firmament, in relation to whom all the others move; and Reichian, post-Reichian and neo-Reichian practitioners are also numerically dominant. Hence I have given Reich and the Reichians pride of place and space in this chapter. However, I have tried as well to cover what Grossinger terms 'the innovative forms now emerging, systems which phenomenologically, improvisationally, regain the present moment, and at the same time pay their historical dues to the myriad techniques and tools developed by their forebears' (1995, Vol. 2: 352). There are certainly plenty of these! And one question to consider as we go on is whether Grossinger is right to suggest that this reflects 'an uninvented cosmology of health' – in other words, whether, in a systematized body psychotherapy, some of these systems would be redundant, or whether the variety of human predicaments calls for an equal variety of creative responses.

All of the forms of body psychotherapy described below, together with some other organizations and centres, have contact details provided in the Appendix at the end of this book.

REICHIAN THERAPIES

Wilhelm Reich

A sizeable majority of body psychotherapists draw directly or indirectly on the pioneering work of Wilhelm Reich (1897–1957); originally a re-spected psychoanalyst, a theoretical and technical innovator who in the 1920s and early 1930s was responsible for hammering out much of the shape of modern psychoanalysis (Sharaf 1984: 72ff). Reich became con-vinced that the internal logic of Freud's ideas pointed directly to the body (Totton 1998), and he gradually began to introduce bodywork into his clinical practice.

This step was thoroughly unacceptable to most analysts, and was only one of Reich's unorthodoxies. He was also at that time a Communist and believed (in line with Freud's own earlier work) that neurosis and anxiety were caused by lack of physical sexual satisfaction, rather than by purely mental stresses. However, Reich developed a view of sexual satisfaction which went much deeper than the ordinary one. He argued that full orgasm, and the accompanying release of bodymind tension, is only possible if we have already worked through much of our bodily and psychological resistance against surrendering to our own impulses.

Exploring this resistance to surrender leads us into the whole array of childhood relationships, and the many ways in which surrender and openness can come to seem impossibly dangerous. Reich suggested that unexpressed feelings and undischarged anxieties are bound into the struc-ture of the bodymind through patterns of muscular tension – what he called 'armouring', which appears equally on a somatic level ('muscular armouring') and on a psychological level ('character armouring'). For

Reich, 'every muscular rigidity contains the history and meaning of its origin' (Reich [1942] 1983: 300), and that history and meaning can be recovered through therapy.

Many later Reichians have agreed about the importance of surrender to sensations and emotions, while downplaying Reich's emphasis on sexuality. Although Reich's specific techniques and observations have often been disputed, his overall bodymind wholism (what he called 'functionalism'), and his perception that the individual's history is written on their body, remain central to body psychotherapy.

Development of Reich's work

Reich's work inevitably changed over his career, and at each stage he found followers who preserved and developed that style of work. It helps to make some sense of the enormous number of Reichian and post-Reichian therapies if we organize them according to the phases of Reich's practice. The first of Reich's body psychotherapy styles he called *Character-Analytic Vegetotherapy*: a rather difficult-looking term which needs some unpacking. '*Vegetotherapy*' simply means 'therapy of the vegetative nervous system', nowadays called the autonomic nervous system (ANS), which mediates the involuntary aspects of our embodiment (see Chapter 2). Reich's work was centrally about freeing our involuntary life from the controls imposed by society and consciousness.

'*Character*' was Reich's name (taken from Freud) for the ensemble of habitual patterns, both mental and physical, with which every person defends themselves against perceived internal and external threat. It is an important concept for many Reichian therapists, providing them with a systematic way of understanding and communicating with a given client's central issues of need and defence (Johnson 1985; Lowen 1958; Totton and Jacobs 2001). So Reich's work at this stage – still heavily influenced by his analytic background – involved the painstaking exploration and unwinding of the client's defensive structures, so as to make it possible for them to surrender to their own bodily impulses.

I have made a detailed analysis of one of Reich's case histories from this period in *The Water in the Glass* (Totton 1998: 108–12). A short vignette may convey some of the flavour of the work – how Reich focused on some crucial detail of the client's behaviour and from it unpacked the whole psychic and somatic structure of their character, and its origins in childhood:

> I once had a patient in whom the central and most persistent character resistance was expressed in a continual chatter. However, his mouth was felt as 'alien' and 'dead,' as if it 'did not belong.' The patient repeatedly passed his hand over his mouth as if to convince

himself that it was still there. His pleasure in telling gossipy stories was unmasked as an attempt to overcome the feeling of a 'dead mouth.' After this defense function had been eliminated, his mouth began spontaneously to assume an infantile attitude of sucking, which alternated with a mean, hard facial expression. During these changes, his head was inclined sharply to the right. One day I had the impulse to feel the patient's neck to convince myself that there was nothing wrong with it. To my enormous surprise, the patient immediately assumed the attitude of a hanged person: his head sank limply to the side, his tongue protruded, his mouth remained rigidly opened. And this happened, although I had merely touched his neck. A straight path led from this incident to his early childhood fear of being hanged for a transgression (masturbation).

(Reich [1942] 1983: 339)

As Reich explains:

The reflex just described occurred only when the breath was held and deep exhalation was avoided. The reflex reaction disappeared as the patient gradually began to overcome the fear of breathing out. Thus, the neurotically inhibited respiratory activity is a central factor of the neurotic mechanism in general. It blocks the vegetative activity of the organism, thus creating the energy source for symptoms and neurotic fantasies of all kinds.

(Reich [1942] 1983: 339)

Here we see the importance for Reich of focus on the breath, a feature of many body psychotherapy approaches. As he explains, restricted breathing is the core of emotional blocking, the mechanism by which we control our feelings and transform them into somatic and psychological symptoms. As well as breathing, Reich focuses on specific details of expression or posture and 'unpeels' them layer by layer, as appears, for example, in his account of working with a young woman whose sense of her own ugliness seemed to derive from a lack of unity in her body image (Reich [1942] 1983: 351–4).

This, then, was Reich's original style of body psychotherapy – something which might appropriately be called 'body psychoanalysis', with a rhythmic movement back and forth between somatic and psychic aspects of the client's process. This elicited a great deal of vivid imagery from clients and from Reich himself, as embodied impulses and perceptions were verbalized and these verbalizations became the basis of free association. A number of individual therapists learned and developed this form of therapy. More recently, some post-Reichian schools have 'reconstructed' it through a combination of Reich's writings and their own clinical experience – in particular, *Analytic Body Psychotherapy* and

Embodied-Relational Therapy. Also, it is this phase of Reich's work which had a deep influence on Fritz Perls and Gestalt therapy.

In this early body-focused therapy, Reich did not work 'hands on', but patiently and gently encouraged his clients to let things happen, to allow bodily impulses to appear, and analysed the material that emerged. However, during the later 1930s his therapeutic style became more forceful and systematic, as he became more confident that he knew what to look for in his clients. He used deep breathing to energize the client's body and amplify the muscular blocks, and pressed tight muscles, encouraging clients to shout and scream in response to the pain to release old emotions 'stored' there. Increasingly, Reich thought about the therapeutic process in terms of *energy*, its blocking and release. In 1945 he renamed his work *Orgone Therapy*, after the life energy – 'orgone' – which he believed he had discovered. By far the largest number of Reichian therapies have emerged from this middle period of Reich's work, in Norway and the USA. They include, among others, *Bioenergetics*, *Radix*, *Somatic Emotional Therapy*, *Integrative Body Psychotherapy*, *Core Energetics*, *Postural Integration* and *Energetic Integration*.

In the later 1940s and the 1950s, Reich became progressively less interested in psychotherapy in the ordinary sense, and more and more focused on powerful brief methods to 'smash the armouring' in his clients' bodies, in the hope that 'orgastic potency' – the ability to surrender sexually – which this made possible would in turn produce the sorts of psychological change necessary to sustain bodily openness. In terms of the three models described in the previous chapter, Reich moved from a Trauma/ Discharge approach, with elements of Process thinking, to a highly confrontative Adjustment approach.

This shift was motivated by a deep urgency about the state of humanity and the world. Many therapists believe, though, that Reich's late style of therapy, however powerful in the short term, does not create sustainable change. Reich's name for the final form of his work was *Orgonomy* or *Medical Orgonomy*, and there are still a number of orgonomists working around the world. The organization which inherited his official mantle is the American College of Orgonomy, which (in line with Reich's own views) trains only medical doctors or osteopaths. There are also other groupings of orgonomists like the Institute for Orgonomic Science.

There are great differences and variations between the different schools of Reichian, post Reichian and neo-Reichian body psychotherapy. Some of these schools, in the inevitable way of such things, are strongly hostile to each other. Perhaps all Reichians of every school, though, would support the following propositions:

- Human beings are pulsating fields of energy.
- Free pulsation equates with health, blocked pulsation with dis-ease.
- Humans are naturally joyful, loving, creative and productive.

• The main factor which impedes free pulsation and natural creativity is the social repression of pleasure, mediated through repressive family relationships.

It would be impossible, and tedious, to describe all the dozens of Reichian therapeutic approaches. What follows is an account of the major schools, together with some representative examples of other varieties (largely those with which I am most familiar). It will be apparent that many of these systems hold essentially the same beliefs about human beings and about therapy, although the terms used may vary. The differences are more about style or flavour and sometimes also about integration of other therapeutic modalities.

Bioenergetics and associated approaches

The largest single school which descends from Reich is certainly Bioenergetic Analysis (more often known as Bioenergetics), founded by Alexander Lowen in the early 1950s. Lowen was a pupil and patient of Reich's and always wrote of him with great respect. However, his own 'neo-Reichian' development made some crucial changes, seen by some as the 'Americanization' of Reich's work. Lowen de-emphasized sexuality, treating it as one important area of human life rather than as the key issue. He abandoned the term orgone, and talked about 'bioenergy' as something similar to ordinary metabolic energy.

Lowen also tended to stand the client literally on her feet, rather than – like Reich – lying her on her back. Where Reich stressed the importance of surrender, Lowen spoke of the need for 'grounding', the capacity to stand up for oneself and move forward into the world. There is a parallel shift from Reich's emphasis on the viscera and autonomic system to Lowen's interest in the expressive somatic nervous system. Rather than working systematically down the body from the head as Reich did, Bioenergetics often begins with grounding and then goes wherever seems to be important.

In this and other ways, bioenergetic therapy tends to be thoroughly active, and at the same time to put the responsibility for change on the client. Rather than applying pressure to tight muscles, the bioenergetic therapist will often ask the client to put herself in positions which stress the muscles further and to breathe deeply, so that painful tension releases as a pleasurable trembling (some of these methods are also used in orthodox Reichian therapy). Bioenergetic work seeks to raise energy levels, and simultaneously to strengthen the client's ability to tolerate and use more energy.

The difference between Reich and Lowen is somewhat parallel to that between classical Freudians and American ego psychologists. Reich, very much the classical Freudian, works from the side of the id, of unconscious desire – represented here by the autonomic nervous system. His emphasis is on helping the ego to surrender to the impulses of the body. Lowen, trained in the ego psychology tradition, emphasizes the ego's task of mastering reality and the role of conscious will – represented by the central nervous system – although he also of course recognizes that a healthy ego needs to give space to the body's involuntary expression.

The well-known American body psychotherapist Stanley Keleman started out as a bioenergetic therapist, before developing his own approach known as Somatic Emotional Therapy. Keleman has made a deep study of what he calls 'emotional anatomy' (Keleman 1985) – the relation between anatomical form and structure and 'the organization and movement of psyche and soul' (1985: xii). He examines in great detail the parallel between patterns of emotional expression and inhibition, and corresponding bodily patterns down to the cellular level. He offers a five-step system towards actively 'embodying experience' (Keleman 1987): 'When experience is embodied passively, the great unconscious controls shape, but a personal form develops when experience is used and digested' (1987: 85). Another 'post-bioenergetic' bodyworker is John Pierrakos, a very close associate of Lowen's who moved on to create Core Energetics, a body psychotherapy system strongly influenced by Pierrakos's own ability to see auras (Pierrakos 1987). Lowen's work has had an important influence on many forms of body psychotherapy, and his books are among the most widely read.

Radix

Charles Kelley, a student of Reich's in the early 1950s, developed a style of work which synthesized Reichian techniques with methods from various humanistic and growth work approaches. He developed ways of working in groups to enable people to recover conscious purposiveness and reconnect with the deep feelings which are blocked by armouring (Kelley 1974). 'Radix' is Kelley's equivalent for life energy, or what Reich called 'orgone'. He stressed that Radix work is 'education' rather than psychotherapy, although many of his followers no longer make this point. Kelley pays particular attention to developing Reich's work on the eyes, synthesizing it with the Bates Method and emphasizing the importance of dissolving 'ocular armouring' – tensions in and around the eyes which block not only clear vision, but also good contact and thinking (Kelley 1976).

Radix is still taught and practised around the world, but like several other psychotherapy schools it has fallen out with its own founder, who now works independently. In many ways it is a very traditional form of humanistic Reichian work, but with its own set of terms, techniques and emphases. In particular, it focuses on the distinction between the energetic 'instroke' and 'outstroke', and divides neurotic structure into three types: the blocked instroke (organized around the emotional polarity of fear/trust), blocked outstroke (anger/love), and blocked pulsation (pain/pleasure) (Pitzal 1999: 33).

Biosynthesis

Biosynthesis is the modality developed by David Boadella, for many years the pre-eminent British follower of Reich and editor of the body psychotherapy journal *Energy and Character*. Boadella's major contribution – drawing on the work of Keleman – is his use of embryological categories to illuminate different aspects of human experience (Boadella 1987, 1988; Labworth and Wilson 2000). He looks in detail at the three embryological layers on which our body is built up: the endoderm, which becomes the internal organs; the mesoderm, which becomes the muscles, bone and circulatory system; and the ectoderm, which becomes the skin and nervous system, including the brain.

Boadella relates these three primal layers to three qualities which he calls 'centring', 'grounding' and 'facing'. *Centring* relates to the endoderm and the ANS and involves 're-establishing a functioning rhythm in the flow of metabolic energy and the balance between the two halves of the vegetative nervous system' – that is, the sympathetic and parasympathetic (Boadella 1987: 14).

Grounding relates to the mesoderm and the three levels of muscular control, the cortical (voluntary), sub-cortical (semi-voluntary) and the spinal (reflex), and involves bringing these three into good relationship (1987: 14–15).

Facing relates to the ectoderm and the various systems of perception, and involves making balanced contact both inside and outside the self (1987: 15–16). Boadella also relates the three layers to the psychoanalytic concepts of id, motor ego and perceptual ego.

It will be evident that Boadella has a penchant for pattern and system (and there is a great deal more complexity to his presentation). The question, of course, is to what extent the patterns he finds are 'out there' in the world, and to what extent they are simply aesthetic – for example, in his constant use of tripartite schema. Mathematicians find that aesthetics and reality come together; and possibly the same may be true in the field of body psychotherapy. It is intriguing that Porges (1997) has proposed a new tripartite division of the ANS, introducing the 'social engagement system' which closely matches Boadella's concept of 'facing'. Certainly, many therapists around the world have learnt from Biosynthesis, which is profoundly attuned to the energetic and pulsatory nature of human existence – at the heart of what identifies a specifically Reichian body psychotherapy tradition.

Biodynamic therapy

Biodynamic therapy was developed by Gerda Boyesen (Boyesen et al. 1980; Carroll 2002a), originally a Norwegian physiotherapist who came into contact with two psychotherapist students of Reich: Trygve Braatöy and Ola Raknes. Boyesen combined Reichian ideas and techniques with others drawn from physiotherapists working in Norwegian psychiatric settings – in particular Aadel Bülow-Hansen and Lillemor Johnsen. This tradition is in fact a whole separate source for body psychotherapy, growing out of the Norwegian convention at that time for all psychiatric patients to receive massage.

In comparison to Reich and Lowen, Boyesen emphasizes soma and de-emphasizes psyche. To Reich's understanding about muscular armour, she adds the concept of 'tissue armouring', bringing out the importance of fluidity and melting: From Johnsen she takes an awareness of *hypo*tonus, muscle flaccidity, equally as significant as the *hyper*tonic rigidity identified by Reich (Johnsen 1976). Hence Boyesen brings to body psychotherapy the important goal of *rebalancing* these two extremes – together with a sense that this is something the body will spontaneously accomplish given the opportunity:

> Biodynamic psychology lays . . . emphasis on the interrelation of psychological process with vegetative process, on the healing force of pleasure, and on the 'dynamic updrift', the intrinsic drive of the repressed libido to come to the surface and be re-integrated. This drive is seen as the bodily aspect of the instinct of self-actualization.
> (Southwell 1988: 180)

At the centre of Boyesen's approach is the role of peristalsis: the rhythmic contraction of smooth muscle in the intestines, managed by the ANS, whereby food is propelled through the absorption process. She takes peristalsis – signalled by gurgling in the belly – as both the effect and the agent of tension discharge via the alimentary canal (what she terms the 'id canal' or 'emotional canal' at the core of the body) and introduces the wider term 'psycho-peristalsis' to describe the her therapeutic project (Southwell 1988: 182–6). Boyesen sees the id as a vertical bodily process and the ego as mainly a horizontal one. Boyesen's theory and practice move fluently between the psychological and the somatic, seeing an equivalence between flow of tissue fluids, flow of libido and pleasure, flow of emotion, and flow of energy. In her emphasis on psycho-physical taking in, digesting and excreting, Boyesen is a body-centred version of Melanie Klein!

The central technique of biodynamic therapy is the 'energy distribution massage' – generally carried out with the therapist listening for peristalsis through a stethoscope taped to the client's belly:

> In Stage I the energy distribution is very much a vegetative massage in which energy is put into the body by kneading and pressure, to loosen up stiffness. The person's stress armour has to be literally dug into before it is released at a bone and cartilage level. Stage II is an ultra-dynamic process in which the massage works from within outwards. From the deeper tissues, by a different quality of touch from the conductor, energy is coaxed on further and distributed towards the tissues in the muscles, and up from the visceral organs, and then eased and channelled into the body's skin-tissue level. In Stage III the energy is gently lifted out of the body's immediate boundary, into the bio-electric field, or aura.
>
> (E. Boyesen 1980: 102)

Organismic Psychotherapy

Malcolm Brown's Organismic Psychotherapy (Brown n.d) is strongly influenced by Boyesen's work in its emphasis on a regulated emotional metabolism rather than on charge and discharge. He uses a wide range of techniques and methods to empower the body's innate capacity for visceral self-regulation, arguing that 'it is the autonomic nervous system, as distinct from the central nervous system, that is the primary neural mediator of the entire inner feeling and metabolic energy flow' (Brown, quoted in Smith 1985: 23). Only afterwards does he involve the CNS functions of will and thought. Brown's whole approach is integrative, seeking to meet the unique wholeness of each client without imposing a system upon them.

Chiron

The Chiron Centre in London offers one of the many forms of highly skilled body psychotherapy, referred to earlier by Grossinger, which have not yet produced an extended theoretical self-description. It was established in 1983 to provide therapy and training in a humanistic, integrative body-oriented style. Its founders were trained in Gerda Boyesen's work, which is still an integral part of the Chiron approach, but the centre seeks to integrate this with Gestalt and psychodynamic approaches. Chiron emphasizes that, whether or not body techniques are used, body awareness is fundamental to its approach:

Chiron psychotherapy is more than the sum of skills, strategies and techniques it teaches. We are interested in grounding experientially – and that includes: in the body – what is often vaguely referred to as the 'quality of relationship', 'intuition' and 'therapeutic presence'. Chiron psychotherapy is characterised by its use of body awareness and the senses as instruments in the therapeutic contact. . . . Chiron psychotherapists use bodywork to encourage grounding and containment, and to support the process of opening to the powerful feelings and conflicts which people learn to repress and suppress over a lifetime. But bodywork is not an end in itself. It facilitates a degree of aliveness in the client and a trust in their own body and spontaneity. Bringing these qualities of aliveness into a relationship – the relationship with the therapist – creates the conditions for authentic meeting.

(Training brochure)

The Chiron approach takes energy – or 'charge' – as a central therapeutic concept, a way to knit together many levels of perception and awareness of self and other in the practitioner. Biodynamic massage is used and taught as much as anything as a training technique, a way to put the practitioner in touch with the reality of body energy in themselves and others; it is not necessarily used with psychotherapy clients.

Bodynamics

Bodynamics was developed in Norway by Lisbeth Marcher, again drawing on the work of Lillemor Johnsen (1976), and emphasizing more than most other Reichian traditions the importance of flaccid, hypotonic muscles alongside rigidly armoured ones. Bodynamics has drawn a precise and detailed map of patterns of muscle development in infancy, correlating the age at which each muscle group is normally activated and brought under voluntary control with the Reichian narrative of characterological development through the libidinal phases. This enables the practitioner, at least in theory, to 'read off' a character analysis of the client through a close examination of their hyper- and hypo-tensive musculature (Bentzen and Bernhardt 1992).

Bodynamics identifies three potential states for each muscle: 'early' (flaccid), 'late' (tense), and 'healthy'. Collectively, these correspond to a resigned, defeated character position, an over-controlled and rigid one, and a balanced position between the two extremes. These three states are applied to each of seven developmental stages between birth and the age of 12 – stages which roughly correspond to the traditional Reichian ones (Totton and Jacobs 2001: 35ff). Bodynamics understands the resigned muscular state as a response to overwhelming stress and trauma. It works with this through a set of techniques called 'resourcing', which have been a major influence on the body-based trauma therapies which I discuss below. Like Biodynamic Psychology, Bodynamics has championed the concept of therapeutic rebalancing rather than attacking the client's defences.

Postural Integration

Within the range of Reichian therapies, Postural Integration (PI) leans towards the bodywork end of the spectrum rather than the body psychotherapy end. It was developed by Jack Painter as a more psychotherapeutic version of the sort of deep tissue (fascia) massage offered in Rolfing. While the work can be gentle, at times the practitioner uses fingers, fists and elbows to grip, twist and shift layers of connective tissue and to reorganize the muscular system, in the process setting off intense pain, and encouraging the client to breathe and vocalize through this process.

Painter uses neurological 'gate theory' to support Reich's model of armouring, presenting the pain of muscular release as:

> a special, transforming event in the nervous system. . . . The nervous system is . . . a complicated set of gates which open and close as stimuli pass through local receptors. What I feel locally depends not merely on the response in the brain alone, but in addition on how local tissue controls these gates. It is as if the gates in a certain part of bodymind were 'set' by a previously painful experience, set by a protective armor which 'freezes' the tissue in and around the muscle. . . . When the practitioner penetrates the body defenses, the tissue is restimulated and the client may re-experience the memories, the events held in the muscles. . . . Thereafter the gates are no longer set by our armor, but are free . . . to be reset for new kinds of integrating experiences.
>
> (Painter 1984: 99)

Together with the Dutch practitioner Willem Poppeliers, Painter has recently developed a more complete therapeutic system called *Energetic Integration*, which rather than systematic work with tissue release emphasizes regulating the energetic cycle and restructuring character.

Embodied-Relational Therapy

The most recent and smallest of the Reichian groupings covered here, Embodied-Relational Therapy (ERT), is the style of work (developed with Em Edmondson) which I myself teach. A synthesis of Reichian psychoanalysis with process approaches, especially Process Oriented

Psychology and also the Hakomi Method (see below for both), ERT emphasizes two themes of human existence: that we are bodies, and that – partly because we are bodies – we are always in relationship to others. In the words of the ERT training prospectus:

> As human beings, we are integrated bodymindspirit; on the whole, we find this condition hard to manage. Our nature seeks to *express* itself freely, while at the same time *protecting* itself in conditions often of great difficulty. This double task of expression and protection makes us often subject to contradictory pulls, and offering double messages about what we feel, want and need; through a relationship which is supportive and non-invasive, it is possible to disentangle our doubleness and allow our process to unfold – which is what has been trying to happen all along.
>
> (Totton 1999)

Embodied-Relational Therapy redefines Reichian work as centred on breathing and relationship. It explores the odd-sounding but fundamental question: *how can I breathe and relate to someone at the same time?* Trying to stay open both internally and externally is a powerful way to explore core therapeutic issues, immediately highlighting both transference and countertransference. This intense face-to-face relating combined with attention to the breath is highly demanding for the therapist as well as for the client. The central focus of embodied-relational bodywork is on re-establishing a fuller, more spontaneous breath – *not* by efforting, but by gradually letting go of our need to protect ourselves from feeling by not breathing. Working systematically through the levels of resistance to spontaneous breath – to 'being breathed' – therapist and client encounter all the familiar relationship issues which emerge through free association, or indeed any other sustained encouragement to let things happen spontaneously and without censorship.

ERT emphasizes the central role of contact in making therapeutic work possible. It studies the resistances to contact which arise, and works with many ways besides breathing of amplifying the client's process, including its expression through relationship, since that process already contains whatever is needed for growth and rebalancing. ERT uses a rich system of character analysis to facilitate communication between client and therapist.

PRIMAL THERAPIES

I am grouping under this heading several different forms of body psychotherapy that all pay primary attention to the healing value of *regression*, the re-experiencing and abreacting of early deep traumas, many of which in their view are structured into human experience. Unlike the next group, whose focus is on specific traumatic events of the client's biography, often occurring in adulthood, the primal therapies focus mainly on infancy and childhood and emphasize events which are inescapable for us all – what we may call *crises of individuation*, the largest of which is birth.

Generally speaking, these events – which also include weaning, the cutting of the umbilical cord, intrauterine experiences and even conception – are not accessible through ordinary memory. Hence the concept of 'body memory' (see Chapters 2 and 3) is particularly important for the primal therapies and many of their techniques are specifically developed for accessing body memories. Primal therapies have been criticized for assuming that 'earlier' means 'deeper', but certainly the more sophisticated forms of this work are well aware of this danger.

Primal therapies have a long and interesting 'pre-history', starting with Freud himself (Laing 1983: 87–93). Among the most important figures apart from those mentioned below are Freud's disciple Otto Rank ([1929] 1993), the psychoanalysts Nandor Fodor (1949), Francis Mott (1959), and M.L. Peerbolte (1975), R.D. Laing (1976, 1983), and Frank Lake (1980).

'Primal scream'

This is the popular name for the Primal Therapy developed by Arthur Janov in the 1960s (Janov 1970), which uses very tough methods of deprivation and confrontation to facilitate primal discharge in clients (including, famously, John Lennon and Yoko Ono). Before and during the three-week intensive treatment, the client stays in a hotel room and refrains from social interaction, TV, smoking, alcohol, and other drugs, and any form of sex including masturbation. Sessions last for up to three hours a day. Janov's techniques have a definite structural resemblance to brainwashing in their approach to breaking down the defences of the individual, who is, of course, willing and eager to engage in the process – overwhelming of the original personality, abreaction, followed by the imprinting of new patterns. This is probably the most single-minded and high-intensity form of body psychotherapy and those who engage in it have often already tried and 'failed' with many other approaches.

Janov claims to have originated primal therapy from scratch, but its theoretical base is familiar from many other forms of psychotherapy and growth work (see the section on trauma in Chapter 3), though unfortunately reduced to oversimplified and exaggerated claims: 'Every cell in our body 'remembers' its natural state. . . . When there is early pain the memory and charge are stored intact inside the cells of the emotional brain centres waiting for their day to be released. These foreign elements are now part of the physiology' (Janov 1992: 25). Janov's tendency to grandiosity and authoritarianism has meant that many primal therapists have organized themselves independently from him.

Primal Integration

Primal Integration is an alliance of therapeutic approaches which have in common a commitment to *integrating* primal experiences into the whole person – body, feelings, intellect and spirit. Primal Integration agrees with Janov that early trauma is the basic cause of neurosis, and that regression and reliving of these traumas can be healing; but it has a more complex picture than Janov of the different factors that need to be in place for this healing to succeed. Regression is followed by the long task of exploring all the implications of what one has experienced. Broder (1976, quoted in Rowan 1988: 31) suggests five phases to primal work: commitment, abreaction or discharge, insight, counteraction (interrupting our behaviour), and proaction (new behavioural patterns).

A very wide range of regression techniques is used by different Primal Integration therapists. These often include breathwork (sometimes involving hyperventilation, see Chapter 3), and sometimes massage and physical pressure. Primal Integration is mainly used by those who already have some experience of therapy and now want to go deeper. Like other intensive bodywork, it often brings up astonishingly deep and ancient pain. However, many therapists emphasize the importance of primal joy and love, as well as pain; and many find that going deeply into primal experiences liberates a new sensitivity to subtle energy and to spirituality.

Holotropic Breathwork

Stanislav Grof has made major contributions to primal integration through his work – originally employing the drug LSD – on birth experiences as shaping factors in our lives (Grof 1975). He employs the concept of 'COEXes' – clumps or clusters of memories cohering around a shared emotional core, for example, around our experience of a particular stage of birth or Basic Perinatal Matrix (BPM); so that, for example, a person who spent a long time in the birth canal may have a whole set of life experiences around the theme of being 'stuck', which constellate as a script or core belief.

More recently, Grof and his wife Christina have developed a form of primal regression centred on continuous deep breathing similar to that of rebirthing (see below), and also using music as a key to emotional memory. Holotropic Breathwork has also borrowed or rediscovered many of the bodywork techniques of Orgonomy. It is a non-interventionist style of work, without a 'therapist' in the traditional sense, and mostly conducted in groups where participants take it in turns to sit with each other and to breathe. The aim is to let the 'inner healer' decide which non-ordinary state to access. Possibilities include BPMs, transpersonal states and biographical replays (Taylor 1994).

Rebirthing

Like Holotropic Breathwork, Rebirthing is not a conventional psycho-therapy, but perhaps part-way between a psychotherapy, a form of yoga and a religion. It was developed by Leonard Orr in the 1970s around a single powerful technique: 'conscious connected breathing', breathing fully in and out in a continuous cycle, without pause, until the breath-ing takes over from conscious control and starts to 'breathe itself', going through numerous changes of pace and depth until release occurs followed by calm and relaxation. Orr found out that this process was very much helped by the use of 'affirmations': positive slogans which the rebirthee uses to counteract negative internal messages brought up automatically by the breathing. A simple example would be 'I can't do it' counteracted by 'I *can* do it'. This has a specific application to the breathing, but is also a general life-script.

Orr believed that the scripts which surfaced were often imprinted at the time of birth and identified the objective of Rebirthing as 'to remember and re-experience one's birth; to relive, physiologically, psychologically, and spiritually the moment of one's first breath and release the trauma of it. The process begins the transformation of the subconscious impres-sion of birth from one of primal pain to one of pleasure' (Orr and Ray 1983: 71).

The bodily correlate of this transformation is a change from the panic and painful tetany of hyperventilation (see Chapter 3) to a state of em-powerment and joy: a breakthrough which several body psychotherapies have discovered, and which many people find is indeed strikingly helped by the use of affirmations. Through using these techniques in the presence of an experienced and skilled rebirther, who may suggest an affirmation at crucial moments, 'the merging of inner and outer breath and its rejuvenating effect become spontaneous and effortless. That is, breathing fully and freely with the spirit, mind and body becomes the natural way for the individual consciousness to function' (Orr and Ray 1983: 77).

The ideology of Rebirthing is that anger and blame are just another life script or 'negative belief'. Hence: 'the client is *not* urged to admit and express negative feelings about parents or to accept that parents had negative feelings about him or her . . . catharsis and abreaction are not encouraged. Instead, Rebirthing focuses on letting go grievances; blame is not attached to anyone' (Jones 1981: 751). On this dimension

Rebirthing, although a regressive therapy, is about as far away from Primal Therapy as it is possible to be.

More recently, Rebirthing has incorporated a striking melange of techniques and ideologies – basically, whatever Leonard Orr has encountered and liked. The focus has shifted away from birth as such and a number of variant schools have emerged. The breathing form is undoubtedly extremely powerful and can facilitate major short-term changes of consciousness; but like every other miracle technique, it seems to need long-term work of one sort or another in order to 'stick'. Classical rebirthing does not offer any sort of therapeutic relationship work to help with this process.

TRAUMA THERAPIES

This small group of 'state of the art' psychotherapies is tailored specifically for work with post traumatic stress disorder (PTSD) and traumatic experience in general. They all draw heavily on recent neuroscientific work in this area, as discussed in Chapter 2 and Chapter 3. Although fairly similar to each other, they vary significantly in how much importance they place on cognitive integration as compared with somatic processing; and also in how far they see cathartic discharge as essential or helpful to the therapeutic process, compared with the potential risk of retraumatization.

Somatic Experiencing

Developed by Peter Levine, Somatic Experiencing offers a set of highly practical and organismically based techniques for dissolving trauma, based on the belief that 'because we are instinctual beings with the capacity to feel, respond, and reflect, we possess the innate potential to heal even the most debilitating traumatic injuries' (Levine 1997: 19). Its postulates are strongly influenced by Reichian theories of body memory and blocked emotion held in the body: 'Traumatic symptoms . . . stem from the frozen residue of energy that has not been resolved and discharged; this residue remains trapped in the nervous system where it can wreak havoc on our bodies and spirits' (Levine 1997: 19).

Levine supports this position with material from neuroscience and from ethological study of animal responses to stress. His techniques have the purpose of allowing the discharge of traumatic emotion while protecting the client from retraumatization – in other words, a repetition of the original experience of overload and freezing. This is accomplished through slow, careful eliciting of memory, with close sensory tracking of the traumatized person's bodily experience. Bringing awareness to their state of aroused anxiety, as it is embodied in breathing, pulse, sweating, trembling, etc., allows them to discharge the trauma bit by bit ('titration').

Somatic Trauma Therapy

Babette Rothschild also bases her approach to trauma resolution on a great deal of neuroscience material (Rothschild 2000). Her method is not too different from Levine's (both are associated with Lisbeth Marcher and Bodynamics), but Rothschild goes even further in emphasizing the importance of a slow pace, of creating safety and a sense of self-management, and also of the therapeutic relationship as a vital container for trauma work (Levine does not work specifically with the therapeutic relationship). Rothschild offers a range of resources for developing body awareness in trauma sufferers, and for using body sensations as an anchor to the 'here-and-now' which stops them being swept away into reactivated memory.

Rothschild's work is striking for its permissive, supportive attitude towards trauma survivors and their defensive structures. For example, she points out (2000: 135–40) that muscle tension – the archetypal negative of the whole Reichian tradition – is a powerful and valuable way for trauma survivors to give some sort of containment to their feelings; and in fact recommends the use of conscious muscle tightening as a resource during therapy.

Sensorimotor Psychotherapy

Created by Pat Ogden, Sensorimotor Psychotherapy is presented as a synthesis of skilled bodywork therapy with the Hakomi Method (see below). It distinguishes between two sorts of problem: 'developmental injury', created from dysfunctional family dynamics that lead to the formation of limiting psychological belief systems – in other words, what psychodynamic therapies would call 'neurosis'; and 'traumatic injury', the product of experiences which appear life-threatening and leave victims feeling helpless and out of control – in other words, what is often called post traumatic stress disorder. This opposition is open to question, and would certainly not be accepted by Reich (Totton 2002a).

The methods of Sensorimotor Psychotherapy differentiate between these two sorts of problem, but also explore the interface between them. Like Hakomi itself, this therapy works slowly, gently and non-violently, fostering an atmosphere of safety in which the client's defences can be examined and willingly yielded, rather than confronted and overpowered. The body and its experiences and sensations are central to the process. Hence, in addressing traumatic injury, Ogden offers:

a method for facilitating the processing of unassimilated sensorimotor
reactions to trauma and for resolving the destructive effects of these
reactions on cognitive and emotional experience. These sensorimotor
reactions consist of sequential physical and sensory patterns involving autonomic nervous system arousal and orienting/defensive responses which seek to resolve to a point of rest and satisfaction in
the body.

(Ogden and Minton 2000)

Although their basic approach to trauma is very similar to Peter Levine's,
Ogdon and Minton argue that 'for Levine, tracking physical sensation is
an end in itself; his approach does not specifically include therapeutic
maps to address cognitive or emotional processing' (2000). To do this
they draw heavily on the sorts of neuroscientific research which I have
already discussed, particularly Van der Kolk (1994).

PROCESS THERAPIES

This group of modern therapies draws on a mixture of very contemporary ideas like Chaos and Complexity Theory, and very ancient systems
like Buddhism and Taoism, to shift the focus from 'states' to 'processes'
(Mindell 1985b: 11–12; Totton and Jacobs 2001: 111ff) and from the
past to here-and-now experience. None of them would wish to deny the
importance of the past, or of fixed psychological and bodily states; but
their trend is to get interested in what is trying to change and grow,
without necessarily asking why this is happening. A deeper interest in
process is a feature of contemporary therapy in general, and more than
one of the body psychotherapies described in other sections – for example
my own Embodied-Relational Therapy – has a process-centred flavour.

Gestalt

Many people – including, in my experience, some Gestalt therapists –
may be surprised to find Gestalt included as a form of body psychotherapy. Yet Gestalt as developed by Fritz Perls very clearly includes and
addresses bodily experience. The classic text *Gestalt Therapy* (Perls et al.
[1951] 1973) is in large part a self-help manual for increasing body
awareness; and the whole theory of figure–ground formation is essentially embodied. As I have already mentioned, Perls himself was a student
and analysand of Reich. Perls et al. take from Reich central concepts
like contact, excitement and even 'organismic self-regulation' ([1951]
1973: 322ff). However, Perls shifts Reichian work very much in a process

direction and rejects many of its trauma-discharge and adjustment elements:

> Reich's orgone theory successfully extends *ad absurdum* the most doubtful part of Freud's work, the libido theory. On the other hand, we are deeply indebted to Reich for having brought down to earth Freud's rather abstract notion of repression.... Reich's idea of the motoric armour is doubtless the most important contribution to psychosomatic medicine since Freud ... In shifting the accent from the recovery of the 'repressed' to re-organizing the 'repressing' forces, we wholeheartedly follow Reich.
>
> (Perls et al. [1951] 1973: 17)

In other words, Perls is not interested in the recovering of past trauma, but in learning to explore the living present – the present of the body and its world. So many of the techniques of Gestalt therapy are focused on body awareness and bodily impulse (and many of these have been borrowed by other therapies) that it has every claim to the title of body psychotherapy. Perhaps it does not use it only because – more cannily than other approaches which include the body – Gestalt has been unwilling to give up its claim to wholeness.

But Gestalt as a body psychotherapy is focused not on discharge and on recovering the past. It seeks to bring the body back to life, back into a constantly shifting and growing capacity to engage and make contact with its own impulses and the world around it:

> People play favourites with their bodies. The awareness or sensation of some parts or functions of their bodies is restricted or placed off-limits and remains outside their sense of themselves.... the result is that these people remain out of contact with important parts of themselves.
>
> (Polster and Polster 1974: 115)

Restoring our capacity for embodied flexibility and spontaneity is of course also the goal of other body psychotherapies; but Perls for the first time sees the possibility of 'cutting to the chase', bypassing much of the investigation of how and why repression occurred and going straight to the question: What process is trying to happen here and now?

Process Oriented Psychology

Process Oriented Psychology (POP or Process Work) was developed in the 1970s by Arnold Mindell, an American Jungian analyst working in Switzerland. Like many of the other schools we are discussing, it is a whole psychotherapy, working equally enthusiastically with all aspects of the client's reality including body process. Mindell identifies a number of different 'channels' in which the client's process can manifest, and between which it can switch. As well as thought, vision, hearing, relationship and the 'world channel' (synchronous events), these include the kinesthetic and the proprioceptive channels – in other words, people's awareness of their movement and body state.

Mindell's original insight was into what he calls the 'dreambody' (Mindell 1988). Body symptoms and other bodily experiences, he believes, can be approached and worked with exactly as we would work with a dream: 'Symptoms are potentially meaningful and purposeful conditions. They could be the beginning of fantastic phases of life, or they could bring one amazingly close to the center of existence. . . . Body symptoms are mirrored in dreams, and . . . the reverse is also true' (Mindell 1985a: 3).

Starting out from this realization, Mindell has created an impressively far-reaching and flexible approach, which uses essentially the same capacious toolbox to work with everything from bodily symptoms to couple relationships to political conflicts. In summary, he perceives people at any given moment experiencing a 'primary process' – aspects of our experience with which we identify – and a 'secondary process' – aspects with which we find it hard to identify and which are trying insistently to enter our awareness through one channel or another. These elements are not fixed, as with the Freudian conscious and unconscious (which confusingly also use the same names with opposite meanings), but are in constant flux as we encounter and move through 'edges' against new aspects of reality. However, some of these 'edges' can become extremely rigid and stubborn; and chronic, persistent bodily symptoms are one way in which our secondary process can make itself felt.

Many of the ways in which POP works with bodily experiences are very similar to Gestalt, although independently arrived at. As Mindell says (1985b: 8), if we closely follow a particular client's process we will find ourselves reinventing every form of therapy that exists! What is particularly attractive about Process Work is its fluid, flexible, playful approach, using some basic principles to improvise effective approaches to whatever comes its way, even-handedly weaving together the personal, the political, the bodily, the relational and the spiritual aspects of existence.

Hakomi

While in many ways a form of neo-Reichian therapy, which places great emphasis on characterology, Hakomi is also very much a process-centred approach drawing from Taoism and other eastern paths of liberation, and taking as one of its central principles 'non-violence'. In other words, the therapist strives to impose no agenda on the client's unfolding process. Another of the central principles is 'mindfulness' – a state of here-and-now awareness without intention which is believed to be the space in which healing occurs (Kurtz 1990). These principles and others are applied to body experience, which is key to Hakomi work:

> Hakomi therapists are trained to track every nuance of the body's gestures, tensions and habits. They then invite the client to study and be curious about these things. . . . The Hakomi method . . . encourages therapists to allow their resonance with another person's energetic qualities to give them clues to the kind of world that person may have grown up in and that they now inhabit. . . . just as the eyes are windows to the soul, the body is like a door that can open to the whole character and belief system.
>
> (Turner 1998: 12–13)

The essential Hakomi approach is to help the client enter a state of mindfulness and then to track with them in a very precise way whatever sorts of experience emerge. Some elegant tools are available for deepening and clarifying experience; for example, 'taking over', where the therapist performs some aspect of the client's process on their behalf, freeing up their energy to do something else. This might mean supporting some bodily impulse or posture, or repeating some internal statement which has been absorbing the client's attention. In its development, Hakomi has seen the therapist as 'sitting alongside' the client, an ally rather than an 'other' (Kurtz 1990). More recently it has been forced to acknowledge the importance of forces like transference and countertransference and to find a place for them in its style of work.

Focusing

Eugene Gendlin's Focusing, like one or two other systems described in this chapter, is not precisely a psychotherapy – for example, there is no attention paid to the therapeutic relationship – but it has many elements of similarity to psychotherapy, and in particular to process therapies. It uses one apparently simple but rich and subtle tool: the bodily 'felt sense'. Focusing encourages the development of a capacity very similar to Hakomi's 'mindfulness'. The central technique is to identify an issue or problem in one's life and to find the bodily state or experience which embodies that issue; then to gently interrogate that 'felt sense' until some shift is experienced (Gendlin 1981). This may involve patiently staying with vague and incoherent sensations for some while, until, often accompanied by a deep breath and relaxation, 'one "knows" what the trouble is. One has not yet found words, but one knows one can' (Iberg 1981: 350).

Focusers argue that the felt sense awareness which they inculcate is a central, though often unacknowledged, feature of all successful psychotherapy (Gendlin 1996). Klein et al. (1969) developed a scale to measure the level of felt sense displayed by different speakers, ranging from Stage One, where someone talks about others or gives a generalized or abstract account, to Stage Seven where 'the speaker readily uses a fresh way of knowing the self to expand experiencing further. The experiential perspective is now a trusted and reliable source of self-awareness and is steadily carried forward and employed as the primary referent for thought and action' (1969: 63). The felt sense begins to appear in Stage Four. A number of research studies since have shown that a high score on the experiencing scale early in therapy correlates with successful outcome (Seeman 1996). Hence one might suppose that a familiarity with Focusing would be a useful tool for any psychotherapist.

EXPRESSIVE THERAPIES

This term describes body psychotherapies which focus on certain expressive and creative capacities of the human body: specifically, movement and voice. Hence they have mainly originated outside the body psychotherapy world – sometimes in an artistic context, sometimes within the field of expressive therapies in general, quite frequently in institutional settings as a form of occupational therapy. They constitute a rich resource for body psychotherapists, a largely separate tradition of knowledge and wisdom about working with the body. (Interestingly, as Roz Carroll pointed out to me, dancers have strongly influenced a number of important body psychotherapists, including Reich, Perls, Mindell, Boadella and others.)

Dance Movement Therapy

As I have just said, Dance Movement Therapy (DMT) has its own set of ancestors, its own traditions and techniques. Although there are a number of older forms of therapeutic dance and movement, including Eutony, Gymnastik, Gindler work and Eurythmy (for all these see Johnson 1995), modern DMT is generally understood to have begun with Marion Chace, an American dancer and dance teacher who in the 1940s started working in psychiatric contexts. Chace described a 'Basic Dance', the apparently mysterious movements and postures which psychotics and others often employ: an 'externalization of inner feelings which cannot be expressed in rational speech but can only be shared in rhythmic, symbolic action'

(Chace 1975: 203), and developed ways to contact such people through joining them in movement. Trudi Schoop, who also worked in psychiatric institutions, suggests that the goal of DMT is 'to bring subjective emotional conflict into an objective physical form, where it can be perceived and dealt with constructively' (Schoop 1974: 157).

DMT has continued to have its strongest presence in institutional settings of one sort or another, but there is also a strong tradition of working in a growth and personal development context. In the USA this takes the form of something of a split between the East Coast psychiatric DMT and the West Coast tradition founded by Mary Whitehouse, with a strong Jungian flavour, taking up Jung's occasional use of dance as a form of 'active imagination' (Jung 1916), and emphasizing the spontaneous and authentic, inner-directed aspect of dance:

> Where does movement come from?? It originates in . . . a specific inner impulse having the quality of sensation. This impulse leads outward into space . . . Following the inner sensation, allowing the impulse to take the form of physical action, is active imagination in movement . . . It is here that the most dramatic psychophysical connections are made available to consciousness.
>
> (Whitehouse, quoted in Chodorow 1991: 28)

DMT practitioners have sought for a theoretical base in a number of different existing therapeutic modalities. Bernstein (1979) identifies eight different theoretical approaches to DMT, including Freudian, Jungian, Gestalt and transpersonal versions. The work of body psychotherapists like Reich and Lowen is also frequently quoted by DMT writers, some of whom argue strongly that DMT is essentially equivalent to other forms of therapy: 'In facing the unconscious dance-movement therapy is an in-depth approach no different from other therapies. It merely employs a different human property, motility' (Siegel 1984: 7).

Hence there are DMT theoreticians who attempt to apply wholesale the systems of, for example, Freudian ego psychology (Siegel 1984) or Jungian analysis (Chodorow 1991). At a deeper level though, DMT clearly stems from an autonomous sense of the role of movement in human life:

> In DMT the therapist understands movement and the way it conveys meaning through its qualities in space, weight, time and flow, as well as its rhythm, shape and symbolic content. This understanding is communicated to the patient both through verbal comments and interpretations, and through the nonverbal responses of the dance movement therapist.
>
> (Stanton-Jones 1992: 4)

This brings in two crucial aspects of DMT which cannot really be matched elsewhere: its close involvement with vitality affect, and its use of mirroring. Both of these do of course exist in other forms of body psychotherapy, as we have seen; but in DMT they are taken much further. Laban's Effort/Shape notation (Davies 2001; Lamb 1965; Ramsden 1992), a specialized language for analysing vitality affects (though this term is obviously not used, being a coinage of Daniel Stern's, 1985), is an important tool for many DMT therapists. A close and precise focus on vitality affect is always found. As an extension of this, most DMT practitioners dance and move *with* their clients, employing mirroring as an initial way to enter into dialogue with them and then encouraging joint and dialogic improvisation. For Siegel, 'improvising is closely related to free association in psychoanalysis' (Siegel 1984: 24).

Stanton-Jones (1992: 8ff) identifies 'five essential theoretical principles' of DMT, which in her view hold true throughout the various forms the work takes. These are that body and mind are in constant relationship; that movement reflects personality; that the relationship between therapist and patient is central; that the unconscious can show itself through movement; and that improvised movement is inherently therapeutic. The last of these is perhaps the most central: the sense that if a person can be facilitated to move spontaneously, a healing process has been invoked.

Pesso Boyden System Psychomotor

Albert Pesso and Diane Boyden-Pesso were originally dancers before they developed their body psychotherapy approach in the 1960s. Their technique (Pesso 1973), generally used in groups, is to start out from identifying the motor impulse in the client and to bring out its interactive element through role play where group members take on the parts of specific archetypal figures. So, for example, if the client yells, hits a cushion, etc., the role players will fall down, writhe in agony and 'die'. The adult aspect of the client is consulted throughout while their embodied self is regressed.

The aim of PBSP then is to bring all of the client's impulses and energy into the fullest possible expression: first of all in bodily activity and then beyond that to bring out the whole emotional and relational implication via role play. There is a strong primal element in the work, as the role players accommodate themselves to whatever the client needs to express and re-experience: 'an opportunity for symbolic rebirth in a perfect setting that matches [the client's] need for expression and personal growth' (Pesso 1973: 8).

Continuum Movement

We have already looked at an example of Emilie Conrad's work in Chapter 1. Conrad (formerly Conrad Da'oud) is another dancer, heavily influenced by work she did in Haiti, who began by working on her own healing from a botched appendix operation which left her in constant pain from abdominal scarring (Conrad Da'oud 1995). The work which developed from this, Continuum Movement, starts out from our 'oceanic origins' and largely fluid bodies.

Through work with different breathing patterns, and through allowing and following the body's micro-movements, clients and group participants are helped to release their 'biped mentality', the experience of the body as a solid fixed form, and recover a sense of the body as 'an ongoing fertile field, containing within itself its own mysterious future' (quotations from Continuum Movement website, see the Appendix). This different felt sense of our embodiment has implications on every level from the personal to the political. Continuum work has proved sometimes startlingly effective with long-term paralysis and other major bodily problems.

Voice and Voice Movement Therapy

Voice plays an important role in many forms of body psychotherapy, from Reich onwards. It is a powerful tool for emotional discharge and often unlocking the inhibitions against using the voice releases deeply held feelings. The voice can be used as a tool of exploration as well, a sort of 'spotlight' which can be aimed anywhere in the body. A number of therapists focus specifically on the voice as their preferred tool. Generally their basic approach is to support and encourage the raw sounds which emerge, and to help the client amplify and complete those sounds in order to relax the voice-producing apparatus – which is ultimately the whole body. It has been said that 'voice is the muscle of the soul'.

An important early figure in voicework was Alfred Wolfsohn (1898–1964), a German Jew who acted as a stretcher bearer in World War I where he heard in the screams of dying soldiers the vast potential of the human voice and developed a method for releasing and training this voice. One of the central British practitioners is Paul Newham, whose Voice Movement Therapy combines these two forms of expressive work. Newham first worked with severe mental and physical handicaps:

> Alone and without a model for what I was attempting to do, I spent many years crawling along the floor, gurgling, screeching, singing and mirroring the many sounds which my clients made in order that I might enter into their language rather than seeking to demand that they speak mine.
>
> (Newham 1999: 9)

Newham progressed to teaching other professionals:

It seemed that my new clientele were inhibited and constricted primarily by psychological issues which manifested in various muscular hypertensions . . . when I was able to facilitate vocal liberation, new-found sounds were often accompanied by intense emotions which in turn produced new sounds as my clients experienced a spectrum of feelings from deep grief to tumultuous joy.

(Newham 1999: 10)

He realized that he needed to understand not only the physiology but also the psychology of vocalization, and as well as theoretical studies he underwent psychoanalysis. In the fully-developed form of Voice Movement Therapy Newham states:

The clients begin by making their most effortless natural sound whilst the acoustic tones of the voice and the muscle tone of the body are heard and observed. In response to an informed analysis of breathing, sound and movement the practitioner massages and manipulates the client's body, gives instruction in ways of moving and suggests moods and images which the client allows to affect and infiltrate the vocal timbre.

(Newham 1999: 18)

As with dance, the work goes beyond discharge into creative performance, creating song and movement from the sounds and gestures released during the therapeutic process. In this way, Newham says 'sounds of anguish can become sounds of triumph, sounds of intimidation can become sounds of victory, sounds of horror can become sounds of joy and sounds of grief can become sounds of hope' (1999: 18).

INTEGRATIVE PSYCHOTHERAPIES

Really, many of the approaches we have already examined are integrative, aiming to offer a whole therapeutic system which addresses all levels of human experience, and drawing on a number of existing modalities to do so. This section though is to provide a home for a couple of approaches which do not fit easily into any of the other sections, and which can stand as examples of the integrative trend in body psychotherapy generally.

Applied Somatics (Lomi School)

The Lomi School in California has integrated body psychotherapy with martial arts traditions, 'synthesizing ancient practices and modern techniques of focusing attention on the entire spectrum of being alive. This approach helps people become centered, steady in their awareness, and full in their heart' (Lomi website, see Appendix).

One of the School's founders, along with Robert Hall, was Richard Strozzi Heckler, from whose valuable and eloquent work, *The Anatomy of Change*, I have quoted repeatedly throughout this book (Heckler 1984). Heckler argues that martial arts like Aikido offer, in particular, 'a way to ritualize our violence and integrate our aggressiveness' (1984: 133):

> Our hopes for a new order are important, but our actions are what will bring the vision into our neighbourhood. Our aggressiveness is as much a part of our nature as is peace. Aggressiveness simply is, and can be worked with in our bodies and minds. Peace, in much the same way, is not some final destination, but a process that we need to work with every day.
>
> (Heckler 1984: 137)

Integrative Body Psychotherapy

The creation of Jack Lee Rosenberg, Integrative Body Psychotherapy (IBP) draws heavily on Reichian and neo-Reichian sources, but also claims to incorporate elements from 'Tantra and Hatha yoga; Freudian, Jungian, Reichian, and Gestalt therapies; Rolfing, chiropractics, and movement therapy; medical models and acupuncture; meditation and dance; object relations and the human potential movement; developmental psychology and work with death and dying; and more' (Rosenberg and Rand 1985: 11).

In particular, IBP integrates bodywork with transpersonal work, aiming to channel the tremendous release of energy which often accompanies the dissolving of bodily blocks: 'When someone has done the groundwork of physical and psychological self-exploration, he will begin to explore the meaning of life and to ponder his individual journey of the soul' (Rosenberg and Rand 1985: 278). Again, of course, IBP is not alone in making this connection: other examples are Hakomi, Holotropic Breathwork, Process Oriented Psychology, and Embodied-Relational Therapy. As I will discuss in Chapter 6, this seems an important forward direction for body psychotherapy as a whole.

A reminder: you will find ways to contact all of these schools of therapy and hopefully to find practitioners near you in the Appendix.

CHAPTER 5

Clinical and ethical issues

Talk and free association do not always release what is coded at a cellular level.

(Conger 1994: 17)

Psychotherapy which addresses embodiment brings with it certain specific issues around practice: issues which either do not arise in purely verbal psychotherapy, or take a different form there. This chapter is intended to identity some of these issues, and to explore them in ways which may be useful both for body psychotherapists themselves and for other people trying to understand how (and whether) body psychotherapy works.

Combining the three models

As I suggested in Chapter 3, probably most body psychotherapists in practice work with a loose mixture of the three models of Process, Adjustment and Trauma/Discharge. The balance of the mixture will vary from school to school and from practitioner to practitioner, but my impression is that most body therapists have at the least some sort of cloudy, perhaps unverbalized image of each model, and that each swings into or out of focus depending on what the client's material suggests. (This seems to be the way in which theoretical models are often used by psychotherapists: at a particular moment a particular client will make us think of Klein, say, or Reich, or Lacan. The better furnished our minds, the better our capacity to respond appropriately to what we are being offered.)

A lot of the time this mixing of the three models will work well enough, despite the theoretical incompatibilities which I indicated in Chapter 3. However, there will be certain points at which the different models actively clash. A simple example of this might be a client with a rigid, stuck-out jaw, whose therapist finds herself wanting to challenge and 'attack' this 'armouring' on a bodily level – for example, by putting pressure on the muscles in the jaw angle with her thumbs, while she asks the client to breathe and make a sound.

Many things might happen at this point, but one possibility would be for client and therapist to become locked in a battle of wills. This can happen even if the client is consciously quite amenable to the idea of softening his jaw! At that point the practitioner might, with luck, ask herself whether she was possibly in danger of retraumatizing the client, of representing in the transference exactly the sort of pressure to conform and 'swallow' external standards which was bound up in the rigidly defiant jaw muscles. She might even yield enough to start wanting to explore without assumption what the jaw was expressing – and might then notice that what the situation required was her own yielding, rather than the client's.

One could invent equivalent scenarios in which any of the three models acted as a useful critique of one of the other two. Perhaps this is the really creative aspect of having all three models in play: that, like the American Constitution, they constitute a set of checks and balances on each other, a way of guarding ourselves against doctrinaire commitment to any one particular therapeutic 'line'. This is the further general advantage of practitioners holding in mind more than one model of therapy; and in the case of body psychotherapy, as I have suggested, these three models seem all to be found in each particular system.

Touching

> In a relationship where passing a box of Kleenex can be ill-advised at certain times, touching the patient's body undoubtedly can create a complex web of repercussions. This is no reason to eschew touching. It means, however, that the therapist's goals and reasons must be absolutely clear and uncomplicated by his or her own personal needs.
>
> (McNeely 1987: 78)

It should be apparent by now that body psychotherapy does not necessarily involve touching. It can be, and often is, carried out with no physical contact between client and therapist. Sometimes therapists will tell clients what they observe about their body posture, movements, expressions and so on. Sometimes they will suggest ways in which clients can amplify or otherwise explore what is happening in their body. Sometimes they will talk clients through exercises and positions intended to develop their bodily freedom, to increase their breathing, or to facilitate the flow of energy. Sometimes they will mirror clients' movements or posture, and this can develop into an active dialogue. And sometimes they will simply consult their own embodied experience as a source of information about the client's process. None of these approaches needs to involve touch.

It is probably true, though, that only a relatively small number of body psychotherapists (Rothschild 2000 is one example) observe a prohibition against touching their clients similar to that recognized by probably a large majority of verbal psychotherapists. Body-oriented practitioners tend to feel comfortable with their own embodiment, and comfortable with physical contact – relaxed and undeprived enough to trust their own ability to hold appropriate boundaries without refraining from touch altogether. (My own comfortableness with touching clients is certainly affected by whether I am receiving enough touch in my personal life.) Beyond this, a number of body psychotherapists regularly use techniques in their work which are based on physically touching clients.

In the next section I will try to distinguish several different ways in which touch can be used in psychotherapy – all of which I believe to be legitimate – and to discuss their clinical function, together with potential clinical pitfalls. In the following section, I will look at the issue of touch from an ethical point of view.

Five levels of touch

Touch as comfort

The most basic use of touch in psychotherapy – whether body oriented or otherwise – is as a way of offering comforting and supportive contact. Many people in our society are starved of such contact. As we have seen in Chapter 2, it has a profound healing function all on its own. Hugging a client in distress, or holding their hand or their head, can be seen as basic human responses, and are treated in that way by many humanistic therapies. One suspects that these things happen far more often than anyone talks about even in the psychoanalytic tradition, where they have been frowned on ever since Freud censured Ferenczi in 1931 for – supposedly – kissing patients (Falzeder and Brabant 2000: 421–3; Grosskurth 1991: 206–9).

Freud's main concern at the time seems to have been about bad publicity; but later objections have centred around the concept of 'gratification', as argued in passages like the following:

> I shall state it as a fundamental principle that the patient's need and longing should be allowed to persist in her so that they may serve as forces impelling her to do work and make changes, and that we should beware of appeasing these forces by means of surrogates.
>
> (Freud 1915: 165)

It is suggested, therefore, that touch offers a gratification of the client's desires which is therapeutically counter-productive: that it offers the client, in effect, a way out of painful feelings which they would be better off staying with and exploring – feelings around not getting what one wants.

Therapy, however, always involves a tension between some degree of 'gratification' (like saying 'Hallo' at the start of the session) and some degree of 'deprivation' (like ending the session on time). The client's unconscious process will create, from this mixture of giving and withholding, experiences of distance or closeness, hate or love, which match their history and expectations. This is what we call transference. As Ferenczi said of his 'twofold method of frustration and indulgence':

> However great the relaxation, the analyst will not gratify the patient's actively aggressive and sexual wishes or many of their other exaggerated demands. There will be abundant opportunity to learn renunciation and adaptation.
>
> (Ferenczi [1930] 1999: 290)

The issue of touch as comfort, then, becomes essentially a technical issue among other such issues, needing to be assessed in each specific instance for its usefulness, appropriateness, timing and so on (cf. Hunter and Struve 1997). In particular, as the Jungian analyst Mario Jacoby emphasizes: 'Most important is the analyst's capacity to imagine in an empathic way beforehand what physical touching might mean to the patient' (1986: 123). Jacoby makes this point in a piece where he explains that he does on occasion offer bodily contact to his clients; and that he does so when the client is so locked away that

> Whatever the analyst said would be wrong. And just sitting silently may be felt as if he or she is not there. It can be an experience of torture for the analysand. Thus the impulse to reach the patient by some direct physical touch seems appropriate.
>
> (1986: 122)

Jacoby also suggests that 'some patients who obviously need body work most refuse it out of feelings of shame, inhibitions about exposing themselves' (1986: 112); and this refusal must not, of course, be overridden.

The central point here is that, just as with other interventions, the practitioner needs to consider not so much what she herself means by the intervention, but what it is likely to mean for her client. The most obvious example is the client who has been sexually abused as a child; what is intended as comforting touch may be interpreted very differently. There are many other possible constructions that a client could put upon physical contact. The same, of course, is true of what the therapist *says*! Yet necessarily we continue to say things, as carefully as possible, and to explore the effects of what we say. In most forms of therapy, comfort is one of the functions of our speech; and touch can be used in parallel ways and with parallel carefulness.

Another analyst who famously was willing to touch some patients was D.W. Winnicott, who did so as an aid to and a support through regression: 'Literally, through many long hours he held my two hands clasped between his, almost like an umbilical cord' (Little 1990: 44; see the section below on regression).

Other analysts, while just as empathically moved by their clients' distress, disagree that touch is ever the best way forward. For example, Patrick Casement (1985: 155ff) describes a situation where a client in deep distress put tremendous psychological pressure on him to hold her hand.

Casement refused to do this, for a number of reasons, which included his perception that the original trauma which was distressing the client involved the *absence* of her mother's touch. For the therapist to offer his hand would therefore tend to suppress, rather than facilitate, a therapeutic reliving of the trauma. It would also, in Casement's view, have given the message that he was unable to bear her suffering and needed to foreclose it. In the end both client and therapist agreed that the real need was not to *be* touched, but to experience him as '*in* touch' with her suffering.

I would recommend that any therapist who offers physical comfort read Casement's argument against this – especially if they come from the humanistic context, where the complexity of the situation and the need for carefulness which Jacoby emphasizes are perhaps not always taken seriously enough. Finally, however, I disagree with Casement's implication that physical holding will *always* be a less creative option than purely verbal and empathic 'holding'. Indeed, Casement himself acknowledges that it is unhelpful for 'the therapist to look for security in a rigid adherence to the usual rules of technique' and that it is occasionally necessary to 'introduce an exception' (1985: 155).

Other analysts like Limentani, however, insist that when 'direct and persistent physical contact has been permitted' the work can no longer even be called psychoanalysis (Limentani 1989: 244). It is an indication of Reich's orthodox analytic roots that he himself tended to see comforting touch as 'seductive' and not to be encouraged (Sharaf 1983: 235).

Touch to explore contact

There is a different approach to touch as contact which is also part of body psychotherapy: that is, the deliberate *exploration* of the client's response. In other words, the therapist might ask the client whether she can put a hand on his chest, for example, and then encourage him to stay with the feelings and sensations that this contact evokes – anything from safety and relaxation to invasion and anxiety. If it seems likely that the response will be closer to this latter end of the spectrum, the therapist may instead of actually touching the client invite him to imagine what it would be like to be touched.

Both these sorts of exploration will of course only happen in a context that gives them relevance, for example when the client is talking about his attitudes towards physical contact. They may be a prelude to and preparation for further kinds of work with touch, like those outlined below; or they may equally well be an end in themselves, a means of opening up important life issues.

Touch as amplification

Touch can be used as a basic method to focus and bring attention to bodily sensations. If the client reports a response in some particular part of the body, then the therapist – so long as it has already been established that touch is acceptable in the work with this client – may ask whether she can put a hand there. This contact generally serves to keep the client's awareness with their bodily experience, and to act as an unobtrusive support for exploring sensation. Here is an example of the use of amplifying touch:

> When she lay down the most pronounced rigidities were around her jaw and neck; she was holding her head very stiffly. . . . I put my hands on each side of her head and rested them there. This had a very powerful effect on her, as usually her head was only reached through words. People made love to her body and spoke to her head. Her breathing deepened and some crying came through, at which point she curled up, screwed her eyes up tight and said, 'I don't want to look, I don't want to look at you.'
>
> (Boadella 1987: 111)

At the same time, through her hands the therapist will be forming her own impression of what is happening at this site in the client's body, using her Intricate Tactile Sensitivity (see Chapter 3) to assess the degree of tension or relaxation, over- or under-charge, etc. The opportunity opens up for feedback between the client's self-observation and the therapist's observation through touch.

Touch as provocation

In some forms of body psychotherapy – notably several in the Reichian tradition – intensive forms of physical pressure are used on rigid muscles, pressing, poking, 'strumming', tickling, and otherwise seeking to provoke discharge:

To mobilize a chronically contracted muscle one must first increase the contraction to a point which cannot be maintained. The muscle thus overstrained must relax. . . . Direct pressure is the usual and most effective means. One will find near the insertion of the muscle a very sensitive spot where contraction is greatest and it is here that the muscle responds best to stimulus. . . . Groups of muscles that form a functional unit in holding back emotions are worked on together. . . . Where muscles cannot be reached by the hands other methods must be used, such as gagging [i.e. retching] . . .

(Baker 1980: 47)

Other techniques used include asking the client to make various expressive movements, such as hitting out, kicking, squeezing, biting, ripping, clawing, pulling, pushing; and encouraging the use of the voice in shouting, growling, screaming and other emotional expressions. This encouragement of expressive discharge relates to Baker's crucial point that 'the muscle will only contract back down again unless the emotion (and ideas) that is being held back is released' (1980). This is what makes the difference between this sort of body psychotherapy and an intensive massage: emotional and conceptual links are being made between muscular armouring and psychological blocks and inhibitions.

Touch as skilled intervention

Many body psychotherapists have available to them a range of body-work skills which they employ as appropriate with their clients. These can include techniques from osteopathy, acupressure, shiatsu, craniosacral therapy, biodynamic and other forms of massage, Body–Mind Centering, Rolfing, yoga, polarity therapy, and many other disciplines. Some of these are taught as part of certain body psychotherapy trainings; others the individual practitioner will have learnt independently and synthesized with their own body psychotherapy practice. We have looked at some of these skills in Chapter 3, in the section on 'Intricate Tactile Sensitivity'.

This sort of use of bodywork techniques is an area of some potential difficulty for body psychotherapy. It raises knotty questions, on which I have already commented, about the relationship between bodywork and body psychotherapy (see the beginning of Chapter 2). What will be the effect on the transference/countertransference relationship of the therapist employing specifically 'curative' skills with the client? The closest parallel with other forms of psychotherapy is perhaps the medically qualified therapist or analyst who prescribes anti-depressants for a client. It would be widely agreed that this sort of intervention has a drastic impact upon the therapeutic relationship, placing the practitioner firmly in role as expert and healer.

In both cases, however, it is plausible that the effect can be brought into awareness and worked with in potentially useful ways. This may in fact possibly be easier with bodywork approaches that, as I have suggested earlier, use a 'complementary' paradigm which may be more empowering for the client than the orthodox medical paradigm.

Ethical dimensions of touch

Thus far I have considered touch primarily from a technical point of view. There are of course also ethical issues involved, sufficiently so to lead many psychotherapists – including a minority of body psychotherapists – to avoid touching clients altogether. The basic argument here is that in our culture touch has unavoidable overtones of sexuality and/or power. Most people's primary experience of touch is either as a child, in a sexual context, or as a relatively disempowered petitioner for help, for example, with a doctor or dentist. As John Conger points out: 'In our culture, people of higher status initiate touch and touch more than those of lower status. Men touch women more than women touch men' (Conger 1994: 13).

Although there are other experiences of touch possible, the entire area is regarded by some as unavoidably contaminated (itself a touch metaphor). It is questioned whether the practitioner can herself be sufficiently clear around touch to use it helpfully and appropriately. Touch, it is argued, will tend to sexualize the therapeutic relationship for both participants, whatever the conscious intention, and may also disempower the client in other important ways. A counter-argument, of course, is to see touch as an active and radical cultural intervention, an attempt to overturn 'the taboo against touching that has prevailed for so many years in psychoanalytic practice [and that] came out of a patriarchal age in which the body itself was suspect' (Greene 1984: 22). However, the 1960s and 1970s taught us to be cautious about the idea that entrenched ideologies can be overturned simply by acting differently.

These are important and relevant questions; and the response of body psychotherapists who employ touch has not always taken the issue sufficiently seriously. Some practitioners simply don a metaphorical 'white coat' and claim a pseudo-medical exemption from erotic response. This ignores the fact that medics achieve this immunity (if they do) mainly through objectifying and alienating the bodies with which they work, treating them as meat machines. The whole thrust of body psychotherapy is in the exact opposite direction, towards a deeper and deeper appreciation of human embodiment. To somehow surgically pinch out the erotic dimension of either therapist or client would be to sabotage the entire enterprise. In reality, such practitioners are more likely to be in denial, which is a dangerous place to be when you are touching clients.

An adequate justification for touch in body psychotherapy surely has to start out from acknowledging that touch between humans does indeed tend very strongly to be both erotic and regressive. It facilitates access to the infant experience of suckling and being held and related to in a bodily way, which is in fact a large part of the reason for using it therapeutically. As we have seen in Chapter 2, what happens and doesn't happen in these very early embodied relationships has a profound effect on how we are able to function as adults. Working with touch enables us to reach back into this infant world in very powerfully effective ways.

In acknowledging this, we are acknowledging our own implication as practitioners in these erotic and regressive fields of force; and acknowledging that this makes enormous demands on our integrity, demands which at times will need every scrap of strength we possess.

Regression

As I have already indicated, the issue of touch is closely bound up with that of regression: the induction of an altered state where we perceive and respond in terms of an earlier life stage than our current one. In the words of John Conger: 'Touch is our earliest language, and capable of taking us back instantaneously to our most primitive universe' (Conger 1994: 13). In this and other ways – in its whole strategy of turning the client's attention to their body – it seems reasonable to say that body psychotherapy has an inherent tendency to be regressive.

Regression has long been recognized as a powerful and valuable therapeutic tool, though a double-edged one. Although Freud was deeply suspicious of the ways in which clients could regress as an escape from therapy, his colleague Ferenczi saw it as an essential aspect of healing for severely traumatized individuals. This positive understanding was taken up by the British analyst D.W. Winnicott, who believed that for clients with a limited sense of self, regression could create the opportunity for 'an unfreezing of an environmental failure situation' (Winnicott [1954] 1987c: 287).

Winnicott's focus was on disturbances of early infant–carer relations, while Ferenczi's was on situations of gross abuse; but it is significant that both men saw touch as an important aspect of regressive work. The work in this area of Winnicott, Ferenczi and Ferenczi's pupil, Michael Balint, is of great value to body psychotherapists seeking to understand how regression functions in therapy, why it sometimes goes right and sometimes goes wrong – what Balint terms the distinction between 'benign' and 'malignant' regression (Balint 1968); the latter being a situation where meeting the client's regressive needs, for example, for holding and comfort, simply generates an endless spiral of greater and greater demands.

One important observation of Balint's which constitutes a useful piece of advice for many body psychotherapists is that the therapist must avoid taking on the mantle of omnipotence:

> The regressed patient expects his analyst to know more; and to be more powerful; if nothing else, the analyst is expected to promise, either explicitly or by his behaviour, that he will help his patient out of the regression, or see the patient through it. Any such promise, even the slightest appearance of a tacit agreement towards it, will create very great difficulties . . .
>
> (Balint 1968: 167)

Retraumatization

The other side of the coin of regression is retraumatization: a situation where the attempt at therapeutic re-experiencing and discharge of traumatic experience succeeds only in recreating the original trauma, and even imposing a further layer of trauma on the client. The client may be no more able now than in the original situation to process their experience effectively. Avoiding this is partly a matter of using appropriate pacing and supportive techniques (Levine 1997; Rothschild 2000), but it may go deeper. Ferenczi encountered this problem repeatedly in his explorations of regressive work and concluded that it was the product of an unsafe therapeutic relationship:

> An abreaction of quantities of the trauma is not enough: the situation must be different from the actually traumatic one in order to make possible a different, favourable outcome. The most essential aspect of the altered repetition is the relinquishing of one's own rigid authority and the hostility hidden in it.
>
> (Ferenczi 1988: 108)

This is an extremely important insight, and one which has been repeated by many later practitioners; for example, Babette Rothschild identifies a group of trauma therapy clients for whom

> developing safety within the therapeutic relationship will take a very long time. In some cases, working on feeling secure in the relationship may in fact be a large portion of the therapy . . . much of the traumatic material will arise within the interaction between the therapist and the client . . . trauma is addressed through the transference the client develops to the therapist as well as the therapist's own countertransference reaction.
>
> (Rothschild 2000: 83)

This is in a section entitled *First, Do No Harm* and Rothschild's whole thrust is against retraumatization, against the use of heroic and dramatic techniques which can easily overwhelm and disorient the client rather than helping to resolve anything. She puts a strong emphasis on trauma clients' need for grounding, for anchoring in the here and now and in their own bodies; and offers a number of specific techniques for this purpose, which are as important for the clients described above as for anyone else. Some of these, together with the contributions of other practitioners, are described in Chapter 4 in the section on trauma therapies.

However, I would argue against separating out a certain group of clients as uniquely in need of transference-oriented therapy. Rothschild suggests (2000: 83) that this group, rather than suffering from one specific traumatic event, have experienced ongoing and systematic trauma which includes the experience of betrayal of trust. But is this situation not the norm in our society, rather than the exception? It may be very possible to do helpful work on symptoms which stem from specific traumatic experiences – often in adult life – without exploring relationship issues in therapy. This work, though, will necessarily be in the nature of first aid. It is more and more widely agreed among psychotherapists of all kinds that work with the therapeutic relationship is a powerful and essential tool for any sort of deep restructuring.

False memory

A great deal has been written about the issue of true and false recovered memories (e.g. Miller 1984; Ofshe and Watters 1994) and I do not want to add greatly to that material; but it is worth pointing out that the issue is a particularly sharp one for styles of body psychotherapy which focus on the recovery and discharge of embodied traumatic experience. On the one hand, it can be argued that 'the body keeps the score' (Van der Kolk 1994), and has an intrinsic claim to be believed, that, as Reich said in a different context, 'the expression does not lie' ([1942] 1983: 171), and that images and thoughts which accompany cathartic bodily processes come, so to speak, straight from the horse's mouth.

On the other hand, it can also be argued that the translation from somatic to verbal levels of experience is inherently prone to error and that, although the *emotional* content of this work is unquestionable, its *factual* content is very much an open question. One example already mentioned in Chapter 4 is the way in which birthing techniques can induce 'relivings' of birth in adults which, while meaningful and useful, are quite clearly not biographically accurate reflections of their births. Regressive techniques used in certain forms of body psychotherapy are not that different – apart from the client's consent – from methods of brainwashing, and may produce similar results.

David Boadella has discovered that the nineteenth-century proto-psychiatrist Pierre Janet, in many ways an ancestor figure for body psycho-therapy, gave a clear and sardonic warning of the need for

> very special precautions on the study and recovery of traumatic memories. The discovery of such memories being important for the interpretation and treatment of certain neuroses, it was necessary to make every effort to discover them when they existed; but since it was understood that such memories might very well be absent, it was likewise necessary to make every effort not to discover them when they did not exist.
>
> (Janet 1924, quoted in Boadella 1997b: 53)

Perhaps this is not such a black and white question as at first appears. Again we come back to the need for awareness that as well as specific individual traumatic experiences – often horrific – there is also a more or less universal *trauma of socialization* which affects all of us in some measure; and that the latter can at times be mistaken for the former, if we come to it with that expectation. For example, in deep bodywork we frequently encounter traumatic body memory stored in the rectum. Sometimes this will undoubtedly be the result of childhood experiences of rape. Often, though, it will have to do with other sorts of violation: invasive cleaning and nappy-changing, punishment for soiling, enemas, surgical procedures – or complex symbolic and fantasy material which has become embodied in this area. As Janet reminds us, it is essential to be open minded and open to the fine detail of what the bodymind is showing us.

Transference and countertransference in body psychotherapy

Working with the therapeutic relationship, with transference and countertransference, is as central for body psychotherapy as for any other sort of psychotherapy. For all psychotherapy, it is only a strong and creative relationship between client and practitioner which allows fruitful work to take place. Exploration of the projections, misrecognitions and fantasies which arise is both the only the way to achieve such a relation-ship, and also in itself an important part of such work. I am of course aware that there are forms of therapy – most notably, the Rogerian tradition – which deny the need for work with transference, and a certain number of body psychotherapists would agree with this. I am personally very sceptical about whether this represents the actuality of their ther-apeutic work; and doubly so for body psychotherapy where, as I have already argued, regression is such an important feature. I suspect that many therapists who deny the need for transference work are in effect doing this work, but within a different conceptual framework.

Relationship work can take on special forms in body psychotherapy. As we have seen, relationship and embodiment are wholly entwined with each other; and damage to relationship is functionally identical with damage to embodiment (Totton 1998). Exploring either form of damage, we are also exploring the other; and body psychotherapists should have the tools to move flexibly between these two perspectives – more than that, to work with the functional identity of the two.

I have argued elsewhere (Totton 2002a) that there is a specific body-psychotherapeutic formulation of the issue of transference, within the Trauma/Discharge model, which is the only one of the three models to use the concept of transference as such. Within this model, transference is equivalent to experiencing the therapist as representative of the 'foreign body' I discussed in Chapter 3 – in a double form: both the invasive, abusive, and/or seductive *external* force, and the subsequent threat from one's *internal* bodily impulses. It is in response to the perceived danger-ousness of these spontaneous impulses and the need to defend against them that 'sensory-motor amnesia' (see Chapter 3) ensues and we lose our full embodiment.

The therapist, like the 'foreign body', appears to offer both pleasure and death. By inviting, encouraging or – in the client's fantasy and perhaps to some extent in reality – *compelling* one to yield to the spontan-eity of the body, the therapist is identified with the early experience of trauma (either specific, or the general trauma of socialization) and with the adults who took part in it, in whatever role. This is a component of all transference relationships in psychotherapy, no doubt, but a particu-larly central one in body psychotherapy.

Another element of all psychotherapy brought centre stage in body psychotherapy is the notion of 'cure'. Probably every therapy client brings the wish to be 'put right'; but the focus on embodiment gives this wish an extra force, bringing in the whole context of what Richard Grossinger (1995) calls 'planet medicine'; a set of practices of bodily healing which no doubt go back to the Palaeolithic era, and of which modern western medicine is a small subset.

In the paper mentioned above, I argued that:

> The notion of 'cure' and 'putting right' in bodywork is a regressive one – a mutual transference fantasy, of great pathos, but negative therapeutic value, which identifies the therapist as a magical rescuer and covers up the trauma again in the act of exposing it. This is just one of a group of fantasies to which body psychotherapy is uniquely prone.
>
> (Totton 2002a: 19)

Although I still find truth in this (see Chapter 6), I have moved on to some degree from the position I expressed there. I suspect that the extreme negativity of this view of 'cure' is in part a denial of unresolved issues of my own. As I said in Chapter 3, I now take the desire to heal and to be healed as irreducible elements of the human condition and of the therapeutic relationship: elements which need to be accepted, owned and worked with in all their yearning, disappointment and frustration.

What remains true in my earlier formulation, though, is the destructive quality of fantasies of cure which are *not* acknowledged and explored by both parties: fantasies that cure can be enacted *upon* the client *by* the therapist, and that cure can be final and unconditional in ways incompatible with our conditions of embodiment. As body psychotherapists, we are often involved in the literal 'laying on of hands'. It is scarcely surprising if this raises expectations on both sides of a miracle. But success in psychotherapeutic terms must necessarily include letting go of such expectations, burying rather than raising our dead and processing the grief that this entails.

The 'laying on of hands' can also very easily accommodate fantasies about the laying on of other parts of the body. 'Sexual healing' is a subset of healing in general and Reich's theories are open to this sort of interpretation, both conscious and unconscious (Sharaf 1984: 18–19). This is both an independent motive for sexual 'acting out' in therapy and also at times an excuse for it. The experience of sexual desire for the psychotherapist and/or the client can be a container for all sorts of forces, many of them infantile and regressive, many of them in effect resistances against understanding and change. As David Mann reminds us (1997: 124), it can also be a container for the creative energy of the work, the urge for a coming together of two people which produces something new and fruitful. It can also, of course, be sexual desire per se, no more (or less) compromised than that between any two people – except that, if acted upon, it is inherently compromised by the context of psychotherapy and the duty of care owed by the therapist towards the childlike parts of the client.

These are issues which body psychotherapy shares with all other forms of therapeutic work. However, transference is likely to be even sharper in a context where there are explicitly two bodies in the room, rather than two talking heads; not that the feelings and fantasies evoked will be different or stronger, but they will be rather more in the here-and-now and accessible to consciousness. As I have written elsewhere:

> Without explicit attention to transference, body psychotherapy can become an hysterical *folie à deux*, either simply replicating the trauma endlessly, or enacting a charismatic 'cure' which is only the other side of the coin from the trauma.
>
> (Totton 2002a: 21)

The subtle and important difficulty with the sort of approach to transference which I have outlined is around avoiding a persecutory attitude towards the client's desires (Ferenczi [1930] 1999; Winnicott [1947] 1987a). When we are working with primal, traumatic material, the issue of trust becomes both central and problematic. Maintaining an appropriate scrutiny of transference and countertransference issues can be experienced by the client as extreme cruelty. In Ferenczi's view it can actually *be* an act of unconscious cruelty, stemming from the therapist's hostility and fear towards the client.

It is equally problematic, though, to veer off in the opposite direction and take everything at face value, acting as if therapy were simply a relationship of consenting adults. There are still a number of body psychotherapists who believe that an assumption of goodwill on both sides is sufficient to facilitate therapy – ignoring our inevitable implication, through the structure of the therapeutic encounter, in the client's traumatized fantasies. The primal integration practitioner, Richard Mowbray, for example, puts forward the concept of Sufficient Available Functioning Adult Autonomy (SAFAA) as a basis for distinguishing between 'human potential work' and 'medical model activity', and argues that in the former 'the practitioner's role is to facilitate, to "be with", to sit alongside' (Mowbray 1995: 183–4). A similar position is taken by Ron Kurtz with Hakomi therapy (Kurtz 1990).

There are perhaps two main sources for this view in body psychotherapy. One of them – the key one as regards Mowbray and Kurtz – is the tendency of humanistic therapy, to which most body psychotherapy owes allegiance, to see transference and countertransference feelings as 'unequal' and politically suspect. This is an accurate criticism of the patronizing attitude of some analysts towards their patients. Unfortunately, however, it leads to a rejection of all relationships between client and practitioner that are not perfectly symmetrical in structure – either between two adults or between two idealized 'children'. Hence bodywork tends to be '*intra*-personal' rather than '*inter*-personal' in its model of therapy – in other words, it focuses on the process of the client, rather than on the mutual process of client and therapist (Spiegelman 1996). This is often accompanied by an appeal to the power of love as the effective factor in psychotherapy; which indeed is the case. Love, however, is not a deus ex machina which solves every problem, but itself an endlessly problematic phenomenon.

The view of psychotherapy as an adult–adult relationship can be found, oddly enough, in Wilhelm Reich, who was himself far from being a humanistic therapist. In Reich the source of this view is very different; it stems precisely from his identification as a medic, a professional offering an expert service. Reich never really addresses the regressive dimension of therapy and often tends to approach neurosis, character structure and body armour as 'foreign bodies' to be dismantled and stripped away by medical-style treatment, revealing the healthy individual within. Our modern understanding is more complex and ambivalent, recognizing both the creative, protective aspects of character and armouring (Totton and Jacobs 2001), and the inherently flawed and imperfect nature of 'health'.

Alongside the humanistic, anti-medical invocation of equality, the medical model itself is body psychotherapy's other favourite way to evade the rigours of transference and countertransference interpretation. This is partly because of body psychotherapy's close association with methods of adjustment. As I have already argued, no rigid boundary can be drawn between body psychotherapy and techniques of skilled physical manipulation. There are forms of body psychotherapy which do not involve bodywork and, certainly, forms of bodywork which do not involve body psychotherapy; but there is also, as we have seen in Chapter 3, a very large area where the two come together.

This makes it quite easy for a body psychotherapist to occupy an 'expert' position as healer, enjoying the accompanying feelings of power and effectiveness; or to use the medical model to stifle more frightening feelings in themselves and their clients. The medical model can even function as a legitimizing container for sexual fantasies ('playing doctors and nurses', 'kissing and making better'). These are not fundamentally different, of course, from positions which can be taken up by verbal practitioners (just inviting the client to lie down, as in psychoanalysis, can set up some of the same fantasy structures); but they are probably intensified by the body psychotherapy context.

These two threads then – the medical model and the humanistic aversion to asymmetric relationships – came together to obscure understanding of transference and countertransference among body psychotherapists. Still in many forms of therapeutic bodywork little or no attention is paid to transference. However, more recently this situation has begun to change; for example, Roz Carroll writes:

> Bodywork on its own can be a form of healing that deepens the client's relationship to themselves . . . Its use in psychotherapy requires a shift of emphasis from the therapeutic relationship as providing necessary safety and emotional holding, to a therapeutic relationship grounded in and guided by an understanding of transference dynamics as an essential part of the work.
>
> (Carroll 2002a: 80)

Techniques of working with embodied transference

Many aspects of the transference/countertransference work in body psychotherapy are covered by the general principles for working with the therapeutic relationship in psychotherapy as a whole. However, there are some specific issues raised by the bodily aspect of the relationship which need discussing. The most important of these is that the client–therapist relationship can and should express itself *between their bodies* and unmediated by language. As the most direct example, one or both embodied participants can find themselves doing, or wanting to do, something physical to the other one: holding on to them, pushing them away, turning towards or away from them, hitting out at them, stroking them, squeezing them, strangling them, shaking them – there is a long list of possibilities!

Generally speaking, there is a need at this point to acknowledge what is going on *in language*. Body psychotherapy gives some specific opportunities for collusion through allowing embodied interactions to remain unnamed. At worst, this can reproduce experiences of abuse which was kept secret and unspoken. However, it is not a tenet of body psychotherapy that such impulses must necessarily be *transferred* from embodiment into language – 'symbolized' rather than 'acted out'. Exploring these relational energies at the bodily level can be powerful, direct and meaningful. Clearly some of the possible impulses at least need to be softened in their effect – for example, it is possible to hit in slow motion, or through padding. Similarly, as in all therapy, it is often better for the therapist in particular to say 'I am feeling like doing such-and-such' rather than actually doing it. But I think it is fair to say that most body psychotherapists would see embodied action *combined with* language as more useful than either on its own.

This is also one of the ways in which a body psychotherapist can bring the therapeutic relationship into focus. If the client wants to hit out, push, pull, hold, etc., the therapist will often offer her own body as a resource for this purpose. The technique is very roughly equivalent to a practitioner asking, when the client describes their response to someone else, 'Do you perhaps feel that way about me as well?' – an active insertion of one's own person into the situation. Body psychotherapy allows this to take a direct and immediate form.

There are other less direct ways in which client and therapist can interact on the level of embodiment. Some of these have already been mentioned in Chapter 3 under the heading of 'somatic countertransference' – phenomena like the therapist developing a headache which mirrors that of the client, or like the interaction of subtle energy fields between the two people (Cameron 2002), so that the therapist can experience the client as, for instance, energetically 'fending them off' or 'sucking them in'. Another interesting possibility is that one person will mirror the other person's stomach noises. It is a fascinating experience to sit with a client while your bellies communicate by gurgling together!

In bodywork as in verbal work, there is a central question about where to focus our interpretation: on the client's unconscious desire, or on the 'transference resistance' which sums up and represents their defensive structure. In other words, do we support the 'deepest' impulse that we perceive in the client – generally, the ego's impulse to surrender in one way or another; or do we support the need to resist, to fight back, to understand the situation as an interpersonal one? This is exactly the question which Reich answered in *Character Analysis* ([1945] 1972: 29ff), coming down decisively in favour of working 'from the outside inwards', interpreting the resistance rather than the 'id-impulses'. In the sorts of terms I have been using here, this is about working through and honouring the effects of trauma and the experiencing of one's own body energy as alien, before engaging with the body's repressed impulses towards pleasure and self-expression.

As a very simple example of how this works on an embodied level, say that a client is experiencing sensations of melting and opening in their pelvis with accompanying feelings of fear and vertigo. It will be much more useful to support and explore the fear first rather than to support the melting. Otherwise we are positioning ourselves in the transference as someone to be afraid of, an ally of the ego-threatening aspects of the client's body experience. We can only consistently take this position when the ego's resistance has been worked through.

Language as a bodily function

Body psychotherapists can be hindered from the work of interpretation through a failure to appreciate that, notwithstanding some of what I have said above, thought and language are not 'mental' qualities which exist over and against the body. On the contrary, in line with the holistic bodymind concept, *thought and language are qualities of the body itself* and separating them off from the body acts to reinstate the body–mind split which body psychotherapy hopes to overcome. In fact, the capacity to think and to speak in language are two of the highest achievements of the human bodymind. As we have seen in Chapter 2, they develop directly out of the conditions of our embodiment.

I will return to some of the implications of this in Chapter 6, but the immediate point is that, although it is true and important that much of what feels painful and difficult in us has its sources in pre-verbal life, this does not mean that it can be dealt with wholly in non-verbal ways. As Richard Grossinger puts it:

> The reason certain problems seem vast and insoluble is that they begin before we have language and they arrange themselves outside of language. Any attempt to heal them must also go outside of language. Unquestionably, somatic therapies do this – that is a big part of their value. But their dilemma is that the way in which they go outside language . . . is not necessarily the way in which neurosis or other emotional pathology was structured primally . . . Then the

way in which bodyworkers voice primal landscapes to their clients requires a fully adult level of conceptualization.

(Grossinger 1998: 98)

The notion that body psychotherapy can actually work non-verbally is mainly an illusion. In order to 'do' body psychotherapy, we as practitioners *talk to ourselves* about what we are doing. We name and analyse and structure our actions and what we are acting upon – a naming which is after all the prime subject of this book! As Grossinger suggests, body psychotherapy cannot meet the unverbalized on a purely non-verbal level. If it tries to withhold from language, it simply replaces one language with another less adequate one.

A better task for body psychotherapy, then, is to refresh the wells of language and thought: to facilitate our capacity to think and speak clearly and truly. This is what the Reichian tradition is getting at when it points out that the brain is part of the body, which can be armoured or dis-armoured; that working with the eyes can improve our ability to see what is going on, and working with the mouth and jaw can improve our ability to say what is going on (cf. Baker 1980: 48ff). The obverse of this is that the same tradition, as Tree Staunton points out, can subscribe to 'a notion of removing blocks in the energy expression without reference to the internal objects and relational dynamics that created and main-tained them' (2002: 59); roughly the equivalent of squeezing out a sponge, then throwing it back in the bath in the hope that it will stay dry. Psychotherapy is difficult enough without rejecting half of our available tools; and this is a message for body therapists as well as for purely verbal ones.

CHAPTER 6

The future of body psychotherapy

The living body is the very possibility of contact, not just with others, but with oneself – the very possibility of reflection, of thought, of knowledge.

(Abrams 1996: 45–6)

By this point, I hope that I have established the existence of body psychotherapy as a credible approach, with its own rationale, its own range of varied and energetic schools, its own body of clinical wisdom and expertise, its own ethical standards, and in general a serious claim to recognition as a valid form of psychotherapy in the twenty-first century. I have also suggested ways in which body psychotherapy has unique and important insights and experiences to offer, which the rest of the field might be well advised to take up.

From this hopefully solid foundation, I now want to explore what may lie in the future for body psychotherapy: opportunities and dangers – ways in which it may grow in authority and status, but also ways in which it might dwindle and become further marginalized. I will be suggesting that which of these futures becomes reality depends in part on tactical and strategic choices which body-oriented practitioners are currently making. Out of this, suggestions will emerge as to how body psychotherapy needs to develop and grow over the coming years.

The impact of regulation

A crucial context for these choices of direction is the current pressure towards regulation and control in the field of psychotherapy and counselling. I and others have argued at length elsewhere (e.g. House and Totton 1997; Totton 1999) that many aspects of this process are pernicious, and destructive of the central values of psychotherapy and counselling. This is not the place to repeat the general arguments. The pressure to regulate does, however, have specific implications for body psychotherapy: a historically marginal and eccentric practice, which now sees itself at great risk of being definitively frozen out of the new orthodoxy, yet also presented with a golden opportunity to re-enter the mainstream at a moment when every therapeutic approach is being forced to make its bid for credibility.

I have already suggested that one possibly unfortunate effect of the regulation process is the choice of name for our ensemble of practices. 'Body psychotherapy' unites us around our most controversial shared characteristic; it does little to describe what we are really about – a holistic approach to the entire human being. In that sense, it actually reinstates the mind–body split which this group of therapies are concerned to overcome, by identifying them with one side of the same tired old polarity. On the one hand, the name 'body psychotherapy' is a bold claiming of territory; on the other, it is the sign at the entrance to a ghetto.

The name in itself is not crucial, of course – many psychotherapies have far sillier names, which have become familiar and accepted over the years. What is important, though, is that the pressure for regulation has considerably narrowed, though by no means yet eliminated, the space for autonomous practice of our craft. Throughout the western world, so far most intensively in parts of Europe, psychotherapy practice is coming under formal control; sometimes by its own organizations and sometimes by the state itself. Increasingly psychotherapists are being forced to acquire academic qualifications, which many see as irrelevant; and being forced to justify their activities in research-centred and outcome-oriented terms which, while often interesting and often productive (as I hope I have shown in this book), are not an appropriate basis for deciding on the validity of therapeutic practice (Mair 1992; Totton 2002b; Young and Heller 2000). The European Association for Psychotherapy, for example, requires its member organizations to demonstrate the 'scientific' basis of their work – devaluing the craft and art of psychotherapy, the way that it is wedded to uniquely personal and unrepeatable context.

Much of this goes directly against the grain of the traditional culture of body psychotherapy. As with other forms of psychotherapy, but probably rather more than most, body-oriented practitioners – when they are not simply exercising their craft – tend to focus on the socio-political or interpersonal aspects of their work rather than on its scientific aspects. Body psychotherapy, as we have seen, has often been explicitly counter-cultural in tone and content; its theories, however complex and subtle, are often not compatible with conventional academic wisdom. (Some of its central assumptions – most obviously, Reich's orgone theory – are conventionally regarded as nonsense.) If body psychotherapy is going to conform to the new climate, its culture will have to change in very significant ways. One may question whether this is a good thing; one may also question whether it is even possible.

Specific versus generic psychotherapy

One aspect of the current climate in psychotherapy and counselling is a tendency to think in terms of the generic aspects of the activity – to consider therapy as a 'broad church' within which differences of technique and theory are of increasingly minor importance. If there are to be large-scale national and transnational organizations in the field, then this generic approach is no doubt unavoidable. But how is body psychotherapy to be slotted into such a scheme? Both its theories and its practices tend to be glaringly different from those of mainstream, verbally oriented approaches (which are of course often very different from each other, but these differences are tending to become elided). If any lines at all are going to be drawn, then body psychotherapy is a prime candidate to fall outside them. And as psychotherapists well know, one of the most effective ways to unify a group is to expel a scapegoat.

One response to these pressures is to try to fit body psychotherapy into the Procrustean bed of generic psychotherapy. This intensifies an already existing tendency to apply external theories and approaches to the field without putting them through a process of digestion. Body psychotherapy is, again, identified purely in terms of its most unusual feature – that it works with the body; and it is assumed that any general theory of therapy can be fitted to this new context. In effect, body psychotherapy is treated as an *application* of psychotherapy – like therapy with the dying, or the bereaved, or children, body psychotherapy becomes therapy with the embodied!

This is to make the same claim about body psychotherapy that Chaiklin makes for dance therapy, that it is purely and simply 'an alternative method for working within the context of any systematized theory of human behavior' (1975: 703). According to this approach, one has only to add 'and the body' to each proposition of the theory in question. Some of the systems which have been applied to body psychotherapy in this way are object relations theory; ego psychology; person-centred therapy; analytical psychology; transpersonal therapy (Vick 2002); and even post-modern and narrative approaches (Turp 2001).

Towards a general theory of body psychotherapy

The approach taken in this book is clearly very different. Body psychotherapy has been shown to have its own theories and techniques, which grow organically out of the experience of embodied relationship. This is not to say that the concepts of body psychotherapy have developed in complete isolation from the rest of the field – far from it, in fact. One can trace in particular an extremely strong line of influence through Reich from Freud's original drive theory (Totton 1998, 2002a). Drive theory, or 'instinct theory' as it is also known, is intrinsically body oriented. It describes how our psychological life is built up from our biological life and also, crucially, how it can then come about that our 'psyche' experiences itself as alienated from and in opposition to our 'soma'. While mainstream psychoanalysis turned away from its roots in embodiment, Reich took up and preserved this side of Freud's thinking.

Drive theory, then, is one of the important conceptual ingredients of body psychotherapy. But it has been absorbed and transformed through seven decades of practice (like Molière's character who realized he had spoken prose all his life, many body psychotherapists do not realize that they are using drive theory!), and married with a variety of other systems and techniques. Many of these are essentially empirical in nature – based, that is, on 'what works' or appears to work; and many are derived from bodywork approaches to healing, rather than from the field of psychotherapy. In recent times, as we have seen in Chapter 2, neuroscience and the study of infant development have offered results and concepts which profoundly support the core ideas of body psychotherapy, and also offer new insights and formulations to develop those ideas. A lot of this has happened within the framework of psychoanalytic attachment theory; but it is not clear that attachment theory will necessarily turn out to be the most effective model in the long term.

I suggest that body psychotherapy – that is, holistic bodymind psychotherapy – cannot work effectively with 'off-the-peg' theoretical approaches developed within purely verbal psychotherapy. It needs its own conceptual framework or ensemble of frameworks (body psychotherapy, after all, is no more a monolithic unity than psychotherapy in general). The existing frameworks are by no means satisfactory or complete – yet; but there is every reason to expect that the exciting work currently being done by a number of people will lead to a new synthesis. What is required from such a synthesis? Here is a provisional 'shopping list':

1 A coherent theory of 'bodymind', which articulates the full interdependence of the two primary aspects of human existence, mind and body. This theory needs to avoid the two complementary errors of on the one hand treating body and mind as identical – which they clearly are not – and on the one hand treating them as separate and discussing their 'relationship'.
2 A bodymind description of human development, which does not separate out the brain from the rest of the body, and which accounts for the emergence from biophysical structure of subjective and intersubjective

qualities. Together with this, a description of how capacities and needs for relationship emerge as aspects of our embodiment.

3 A new vocabulary which brings together drive and attachment theories into a single whole, centred around the role of pleasure and security in providing a developmental matrix, and the strategies and tactics which human beings used to deal with the deprivation of pleasure and security. A starting point here would be Reich's statement that: 'On an elementary level, there is but one desire which issues from the biopsychic unity of the person, namely the desire to discharge inner tensions . . . This is impossible without contact with the outer world. Hence, the *first* impulse of *every* creature must be the desire to establish contact with the outer world' (Reich [1945] 1972: 271, original italics)

4 An adequate language for discussing vitality affect/affective style/ embodied character. (Laban notation could be an important element in this.) Linked with this, a fully worked-out theory of body energy which both distinguishes and articulates the relationship between biophysical energy and vitality affect.

5 The development out of all the above of a set of technical tools and guidelines for clinical work, centred on the facilitation of embodied relationship.

This is clearly an ambitious project. But it should be apparent from this book as a whole that many elements of the above are already in place, or nearly so. There is a sense that we are trembling on the edge of a new paradigm for body psychotherapy – which will, if achieved, become the most adequate paradigm for psychotherapy as a whole, since it will incorporate a far greater area of human experience. What is needed above all is a new vocabulary – one which owes no allegiance to any one model from the past. The difficulty is that vocabularies cannot be created out of whole cloth. The transition from a 'pidgin', an artificial mixture of languages, to a 'creole', a genuine new tongue, is something which unavoidably takes time.

Rattling and shaking body psychotherapy

As a contribution to this potential new synthesis, it is important to look at the existing state of play in body psychotherapy with a fresh and critical eye, to identify what is fossilized and needs to be junked or renewed. There is a tradition in humanistic work of something called 'rattling and shaking': a process of friendly but robust challenge, which opens up and confronts the habits and assumptions of the individual or group in question. In what follows I want to place body psychotherapy under this sort of scrutiny; not in order to knock it down, but to help it stand more firmly.

One of the most incisive challenges to psychotherapy which I have encountered is Adam Phillips's observation that 'we can usefully ask of any psychoanalytic theory' – or equally, any psychotherapeutic theory – 'what wishes it tries to satisfy' (1994: 100–1). What, in other words, are the unconscious motivations behind the theory? What anxiety would it lift, what aspect of human existence would be easier, if it were to be true? To answer this question is of course not to disprove the theory – sometimes wishes do come true; but it does encourage us to step back and question critically what non-rational motives may have led us to accept the theory's reality.

The example which immediately comes to mind from the body psychotherapy tradition is Wilhelm Reich's orgasm theory – that the capacity for full orgasm is functionally identical with psychosomatic health. It seems very plausible that the wish being satisfied here is the wish that the moment of sexual bliss and relaxation could become permanent: the wish, in fact, for satisfaction itself. More deeply, one could say, the wish is for *sexual healing* – a wish very widely encoded into body psychotherapy, and itself only one version of the more general wish for cure with which, it seems to me, body psychotherapy constantly dialogues. This in fact has emerged as one of the ongoing themes of this book: the problematic, often paradoxical, nature of healing, of cure.

Within the body psychotherapy tradition we encounter on the one hand a triumphant, milleniarist vision of what we might call the 'perfect body', the body stripped of all its cultural and familial chains and stains, the body cleansed and renewed by a therapeutic last trump and restored to its full capacity for pleasure, truth and creativity. On the other hand, we find a more difficult and compromised acknowledgement of the body in at least partial defeat – by trauma, by socialization, by ageing and illness and injury, by the drag of gravity itself; a perception that total cure, absolute healing, are fantasies not realistic goals, part of the problem rather than part of the solution; and emerging from all this, a practice of accommodation, acceptance and indeed love for the body's panoply of protective self-distortions.

Each of these viewpoints can function as a closed posture, a fixed commitment to either starry optimism or hard-bitten pessimism. Used in this way, both are therapeutically destructive. The former reaches its apogee in New Age body fascism; the latter, in styles of work which try to achieve 'adjustment', to fold the client's bodymind away into the cramped space and shape allowed to it by cultural norms. Actually, of course, both strategies amount to the same thing. Applied as universal realities, both try to fit the client to the therapy rather than vice versa. Both world views are of great usefulness when they operate as *moments* in the therapeutic process; when they can take up and articulate and support – or equally, confront and challenge – the corresponding aspect of the client, the optimism and pessimism embodied in each of us through the inherent structure of coming-to-being as a bodymind, the need at one moment to bow to reality and at the next moment to contest it.

The optimistic strand of body psychotherapy, however, can quite easily become a malignantly charismatic performance of cure, where whatever symptomatic improvement is achieved (and this may be quite dramatic) masks an underlying reinforcement of neurotic patterns. Richard Grossinger argues this strongly:

> Unless one breaks into their own internal dialogue, the best somatic treatments become incorporated into ancient dialogues such that, as they improve some visceral, neuromuscular, or psychospiritual condition, they also amplify core neurosis – the gap between the languaging self that is mature and cerebral and the primitive self that is still thrashing about . . . Unless a therapist – including a somatic therapist – takes into account the way voices, compulsions and neuroses are built and layered into the psyche, he or she is merely fantasizing emotional work parallel to somatic work.
>
> (Grossinger 1998: 103)

Body psychotherapy has long been haunted by charismatic performers – sometimes actively abusive, but more often sincerely misguided hunters after cure, the unachievable 'perfect body' of unconscious desire. Not surprisingly, such charismatic lineages are actively uninterested in analysing what goes on in their work; faced with criticism, or even questioning, they have tended to reach for handy shotgun diagnoses like 'emotional plague character' or 'intellectual defence' (more pithily, 'head trip').

Does body psychotherapy 'work'?

The previous section should make clear that the problematic element in this question is the idea of 'working' itself. This is an issue for the whole of psychotherapy, of course. In the era of regulation and 'value for money', it creates repeated clashes between different notions of what 'working' is; for example, between those who see the purpose of psychotherapy as helping people to function in their environment as it is, and those who see its purpose as enabling people to find the courage to identify and question what is toxic in their current environment.

Body psychotherapy has from its inception carried the fantasy of what I have called the 'perfect body' – what Reich called the 'genital character', not dissimilar from what others call an 'enlightened being'. Charles Kelley, who was part of the group around Reich in the 1950s, is in no doubt that those claiming to be 'genital characters' were as imperfect as the next person (personal communication). As Marvin Spiegelman wrote to me:

Reichian work (eight years of it!) surely opened up the energy dimension for me. After the first few years, I would spend the end of the session in a kind of energy bliss, which would revolve into armor again within a few hours. But that was the source of Reich's pessimism, wasn't it?

(Spiegelman, personal communication)

This refers to the fact that Reich himself, the quintessentially millenial optimist of body psychotherapy, fell finally into deep despair about the possibility of achieving lasting therapeutic change in adults, and saw hope only in a combination of social and educational action with protecting the unarmoured energy of infants and children (Mann and Hoffman 1990: 86; Sharaf 1983: 318ff). Yet Reich's final pessimism was perhaps only a function of his grandiose optimism. Only because his goals were so high did he see himself as failing so profoundly.

It would be sad, though, to see body psychotherapy lower its sights too far and perhaps restrict itself to a gentle amelioration of the suffering caused by psychosocial conditions. Body psychotherapy has always had a radical edge, a stark awareness of how what I have called the trauma of socialization impacts individuals. This may lead it to aspire further than it can reach; but that is surely preferable to settling for less than enough. If a large proportion of the problems we see in the therapy room do indeed have social causes, then we surely need to say so – while at the same time helping clients, not only to endure their conditions, but also to modify them.

On the more mundane level of 'working', as we saw in Chapter 1, there is only anecdotal evidence. This familiar phrase, though, can be misleading! 'Anecdotal evidence' means real people bearing witness as to how body psychotherapy has helped them live richer and more satisfying lives. Such evidence as we have suggests that body psychotherapy is experienced by clients as useful to much the same (rather high) extent as other forms of psychotherapy. It would be valuable, though, to construct further research programmes into what body psychotherapy can do, and how it does it.

Putting the 'mind' back in 'bodymind'

All the above discussion connects with the historical tendency of body psychotherapy to take an unreflective, anti-intellectual stance towards its own theory and practice. Through the sort of misconception which I have already outlined, work with or through the body has at times become identified *over and against* work with or through the mind. This attitude takes up and generalizes Reich's portrayal of empty verbalism as a therapeutic defence:

In many cases the function of speech has deteriorated to such a degree that the words express nothing whatever and merely represent a continuous, hollow activity on the part of the musculature of the neck and the organs of speech. . . . It is my opinion that in many psychoanalyses which have gone on for years the treatment has become stuck in this pathological use of language.

(Reich [1945] 1972: 360–1)

Reich's critique of empty pseudo-intellectualism has been turned into a critique of thinking per se (a highly inappropriate use of such an intellectual heavyweight as Reich himself); so that in some quarters body psychotherapy became a muscular cult of action rather than articulation. Hence Baker's sustained attack on the liberal intellectual (1967: 170ff) and the general idealization of 'the truth of the body' which I discussed at the end of Chapter 2.

This phase in the history of body psychotherapy seems to be over. A new generation of practitioners fully recognizes the identity, rather than the opposition, of body and mind, and gives a proper place to thinking and speaking, both in clinical practice and in the conceptualization of bodymind psychotherapy in all its complexity. This leads to a critical revaluation of many of the traditional elements of body psychotherapy's self-description; in particular, the elements which derive from bodywork practices.

There are many questions still to be answered here. Some of the concepts dealt with in verbal psychotherapies are not easy to translate into embodiment terminology. How, for example, does ambivalence express itself on a bodily level? What exactly is the bodily equivalent of projection? There may not yet be answers to these questions, but they are at least being asked – and with acknowledgement of the possibility that body psychotherapy may even be able to critique or modify some of these concepts.

Subtle and spiritual bodies

Man has no body distinct from his soul.
(William Blake, *The Marriage of Heaven and Hell*)

As well as the opposition we have already discussed between body and mind, western culture tends strongly to posit an opposition between body and soul or spirit. The assumption is often made that to value the body means to devalue the spirit, and vice versa: that a focus on bodily experience is 'materialist', understood either positively or negatively but in either case as anti-spiritual. Much the same goes for those areas of experience which come under such titles as 'psychic', 'paranormal', 'subtle energy', and so on.

Csordas quotes a wonderful and illuminating dialogue between an anthropologist and an indigenous inhabitant of New Caledonia.

> Leenhardt suggested that the Europeans had introduced the notion of 'spirit' to the indigenous way of thinking. His interlocutor contradicted him, pointed out that they had 'always acted in accord with the spirit. What you've brought us is the body.'
> (Csordas 1994: 6, quoting Leenhardt [1947] 1979: 164)

Among other things this points up one of the potential pitfalls of body psychotherapy: that it could end up 'bringing us the body' as something without spirit, something distinct from spirit rather than the immanent expression of spirit. William Blake makes the same point in the epigraph to this section: not that there is no soul separate from the body, but that there is no body separate from the soul.

Apart, oddly enough, from Reich himself, who always identified himself firmly (and against all the evidence) as a materialist scientist, and passionately opposed what he called 'mysticism' (Mann and Hoffman 1990: 181ff), it would probably be hard to find a body psychotherapist who agreed with the traditional western picture of 'body vs. spirit'. The experience of many, many body psychotherapy trainees and clients has been exactly the opposite: that the more deeply one goes into the experience of embodiment, the more strongly one becomes aware of the spiritual and subtle aspects of reality.

This is not primarily a theoretical process, but an experiential one. Body psychotherapy, it seems, cleanses the 'doors of perception' which Blake and Aldous Huxley describe. It facilitates the courage to perceive and accept what *is*, rather than what is supposed to be; and this turns out to be 'not only queerer than we suppose, but queerer than we *can* suppose' (J.B.S. Haldane, quoted in Partington 1996: 321). Body psychotherapy offers experiences which can be conceptualized as past lives, disembodied spirits, fairies, earth and cosmic energies, telepathy, clairvoyance, synchronicity, Spirit, God. Depending on character type, some people talk loudly about these experiences, while others keep quiet. (Body psychotherapy as a discipline tends to keep quiet about it these days, as part of its strategy for acceptance.) Effective body psychotherapy can not only open up our perception of these levels of reality, but can also create the groundedness to tolerate such perception without psychosis, without losing the capacity to operate in the consensual everyday world (see the discussion of 'grounding' and 'skying' in Chapter 3).

In this way, body psychotherapy has something important to offer the myriad spiritual and psychic disciplines: a firm anchor in embodiment. The opposite polarity to crude materialism is a devaluing and rejection of the body, which treats incarnation as something approaching a punishment rather than an opportunity. As Richard Strozzi Heckler reminds us:

If our longing for experience of union is not grounded in the lived experience of the body, we begin to evade responsibility, commitment, and intimacy. To separate our bodily life from our spiritual life is a way of artificially separating from life itself.

(Heckler 1984: 112)

There are elements of body psychotherapy which strongly resemble spiritual practice; for example breathwork, which is in many ways a form of meditation. Spiritual traditions often focus on the breath; the word 'spirit' itself means 'breath', the breath of life. As mentioned in Chapter 3, the breath is also a point of interface between the voluntary and involuntary aspects of existence, between will and spontaneity. Hence surrender to breathing is surrender to the non-egoic. Freud and Reich both make it clear that the ego, as a restrictive illusion of control and unity, can in many ways be identified with chronic muscular tension (Freud 1923: 364; Reich [1942] 1983: 299ff). Body psychotherapy facilitates the release of these patterns of tension and hence dissolution of the 'spastic I' (Totton 1998: 105). Many experiences can emerge through breathwork which are also found in explicitly spiritual practices.

An interesting sidelight on all this is that Israel Regardie, a ritual magician who was at one time Aleister Crowley's secretary, later became a Reichian therapist practising in Los Angeles. Marvin Spiegelman, a well-known Jungian analyst, spent some time in therapy with Regardie and has written an account of his experience (Spiegelman 1992). Regardie recommended that aspiring magicians go through Reichian body psychotherapy in order to open up their capacity to sense subtle energies; and for some while I had a trickle of clients coming for this reason.

The Dead White Male factor

One further piece of 'rattling and shaking' is important. Like most forms of psychotherapy, body psychotherapy can be fairly parochial in its viewpoint. Many of its central figures are, in simple fact, dead white Middle European males; and there are aspects of its theory and practice which are open to critique as relevant mainly to white, middle-class First Worlders. Certainly body psychotherapists tend to make generalizations – about character types, patterns of armouring and the value of emotional expressiveness – which may well not be of universal application. There are some versions of character theory, for example (Baker 1980; Eiden 2002), which assume an essential rather than a socially conditioned link between the so-called 'hysteric' character and women and between the so-called 'phallic' character and men.

Body psychotherapy can be used in deeply conservative ways, because conditioned bodily habits and perceptions can *appear* to us as simple and absolute truths rather than as socially imposed phenomena. A body psychotherapy which goes behind these appearances – as all psychotherapies must surely strive to do – could address both universal human similarities (we all have bodies, which are all pretty much the same), and specific human differences like gender, ethnicity and age; as well as the different *uses of the body* which respond to specific sociocultural conditions, or which simply express the range of human creativity. Such a body psychotherapy, however, would have to recognize and respond to all the ways in which difference is turned into inequality. Most oppression of particular human subgroups has been based on aspects of the body, because they are characteristics which are very hard to disguise or alter – gender, ethnicity, age, etc.

Odd body out

Such a body psychotherapy might well resemble a new shamanism. Shamanic elements are apparent in body psychotherapy as it already exists (Grossinger 1995) – Reich, for example, believing himself to be a rational scientist, found himself working to make rain and performing what were essentially alchemical experiments (Sharaf 1984: 370ff). Another important body psychotherapist, Arnold Mindell, has written *The Shaman's Body: A New Shamanism for Transforming Health, Relationships, and the Community* saying that:

> Indigenous teachers have taught me that the quality of life depends upon body sensations that are linked to the environment, to what I call the shaman's body. According to medicine people living in native settings around the world, and to mystical traditions, the shaman's dreamingbody, when accessed, is a source of health, personal growth, good relationships, and a sense of community.
>
> (Mindell 1993: 3)

These ideas and others like them point the way for a unitary body-mindspirit therapy which is also socially transformative. The Jungian analyst McNeely offers a parallel vision of a future for psychotherapy in which:

> Analysts who are used to thinking in terms of mental structures and mental mechanisms of defense will learn to conceptualize in terms of the subtle body and freeing blockages in the somatic unconscious. Their aim will be to create an energy-body of substance which can express the fullest manifestation of Self. Just as we now see psychosomatic processes in physical and mental-emotional images, so will we be able to visualize and sense kinesthetically what is

occurring in the body of the analysand, and this will be our automatic and natural response, We will see consciousness fill out spatially within and beyond the physical body as individuation takes place and is expressed in the subtle body or dreambody.

(McNeely 1987: 107)

It is at least as easy, unfortunately, to envision a thoroughly dystopic future in which the body is increasingly devalued, controlled, regulated and separated from its animal heritage through a mixture of biochemical and cybernetic interventions. There are already those who enthusiastically imagine the abandonment of the human body altogether, and our transformation into computer intelligences or cyborg entities. Certainly these imaginings represent our cultural alienation from the body; but it is an alienation which technology will soon be able to instantiate literally.

In any such future there could be little public place for body psychotherapy – although such changes would surely be as uneven and contested as any other social developments, and some form of body psychotherapy would no doubt survive in the margins and interstices. But part of the immediate future for body psychotherapy, I would suggest – both on the micro-level of individual therapy and the macro-level of public forums – is precisely to oppose the social forces which are carrying us in this sort of direction, and to articulate the reasons why they need to be opposed. This may imply (and I write this in all sympathy for practitioners who are rightly proud of their work and want proper recognition for it) that bodymind psychotherapy stops seeking a mainstream acceptance which may well be unattainable and acknowledges fully its own status as 'odd one out', both in the world of psychotherapy and in the world in general.

Many of the difficulties in integrating bodymind psychotherapy into psychotherapy as a whole are reflections of general cultural problems around bodies and touch. Body-centred therapy rubs – literally – on some of society's sorest spots. It brings to light all the ways in which themes and experiences of embodiment become traumatizing aspects of individual history, through our culture's deep sickness in relation to sexuality. Child sexual abuse is the most obvious example of this; but as I have been arguing throughout this book, we are *all* traumatized through our adaptation to society's rules about sexuality, pleasure and body regulation, as these rules are mediated through the family.

Working with and through the body, and with and through the feelings and thoughts that this work mobilizes, necessarily uncovers our trauma of socialization: a trauma which cannot fully be repaired or undone. To fantasize such an undoing is to fantasize a state outside culture. Yet each culture has specific conditions and qualities and these are open to change, however difficult and gradual. The practice and theory of body psychotherapy, I would argue, implies that our culture needs to create more space within itself for *embodied pleasure* – not the trivial enjoyments and titillations which surround us, but a deep pleasure grounded in infant experiences of safety and nurturing, pleasure which is identified with the capacity for achievement and intimate relationship. One of Reich's sayings has been and remains important for me: 'Love, work and knowledge are the wellsprings of existence. They should also govern it' (Reich 1960: epigraph). This makes no direct reference to the body; but it grows out of the ground of body psychotherapy, and in my view expresses its deepest aspirations. Reich also said that 'human culture does not exist yet' (Reich [1948] 1967: 100). Body psychotherapy may help to create it.

APPENDIX

Resources

This section should enable readers to make contact with practitioners and organizations for all the forms of body psychotherapy mentioned in this book. I have tried to include contact addresses from a range of different countries from international to local, but some persistence may be needed to find resources in particular areas. Organizations which offer training in body psychotherapy are marked with an asterisk (*).

Umbrella bodies

European Association for Body Psychotherapy
EABP Secretariat
Jill van der Aa
Leidsestraat 106–108/2
1017 PG Amsterdam
Netherlands
Tel: +31 20 330 2703
Fax: +31 20 625 7312
email: eabpsecretariat@planet.nl
www.eabp.org/

US Association for Body Psychotherapy
7831 Woodmont Avenue
Suite 294
Bethesda
Maryland 20814
USA
Tel: +1 202 466 1619

Fax: +1 212 629 2039
email: usabp@usabp.org
www.usabp.org/

Reichian, neo- and post-Reichian therapies

Reichian/Orgone therapists – a listing of those who have sent in or posted
information of their service, listed by country and location within country:
www.orgone.org/therpy00.htm

Analytic body psychotherapy

Guy Gladstone
The Open Centre
188 Old Street
London EC1V 9FR
UK
Tel: +44 (0)20 7272 6672

Biodynamic psychotherapy

Institute of Biodynamic Psychology and Psychotherapy*
126 Rainville Court
Rainville Road
London W6 9HJ
UK
Tel: +44 (0)20 7381 9075
Fax: +44 (0)20 7381 6110
email: ibpp@biodynamic.org
www.biodynamic.org/

London School of Biodynamic Psychotherapy*
Willow Cottage
off Wokingham Road
Hurst
Berkshire RG10 0RU
UK
Tel: +44 (0)7000 794 725
email: enquiries@lsbp.org.uk
www.lsbp.org.uk

Bioenergetics

Institute of Bioenergetic Analysis*
155 Main Street
Suite 304
Brewster
NY 10509
USA

Tel: +1 845 279 8474
Fax: +1 845 279 8402
email: IIBANET@aol.com
www.bioenergetic-therapy.com/

European Federation for Bioenergetic Analysis-Psychotherapy
Dr Massimo Marietti
Via Novara 139
20153 Milano
Italy
Tel: +39 0240 910915
Fax: +39 0240 910915
email: mariettm@tin.it
www.digilander.iol.it/biopsy/efbap/

Gentle Bioenergetics Foundation
Richard C. Overly
29 Lovers Loop Road
Asheville
NC 28803
USA
Tel: +1 828 298 5454
email: rcoverly@gentlebio-energetics.com
www.gentlebio-energetics.com/

Biosynthesis

International Institute for Biosynthesis*
Benzenrüti 6
CH-9410 Heiden
Switzerland
Tel: +41 (0)71 891 68 55
Fax: +41 (0)71 891 58 55
email: biosynthesis@bluewin.ch
www.biosynthesis.org/

Instituto Brasileiro de Biossíntese*
Rua Pascoal Vita 682
Cep 05445-001
São Paulo
Brazil
Tel: +55 11 8703221/8700315
email: rkignel@u-netsys.com.br

Mark Ludwig
PO Box 713
New Paltz
NY 12561
USA
email: MaLud123@aol.com

Bodynamics

Bodynamic International ApS*
Struenseegade 13A
2200 København N
Denmark
Tel: +45 35 35 43 21
Fax: +45 35 35 06 45
email: bodynamic@bodynamic.dk
www.bodynamic.dk/

Bodynamic Institute USA*
PO Box 1708
Novato
CA 94948
USA
Tel: +1 415 258 4805
email: info@bodynamicusa.com
www.bodynamicusa.com/

Bodynamic Canada*
3026 Arbutus Street
Vancouver
BC V6J 4P7
Canada
Tel: +1 604 878 7660
email: info@bodynamic.ca
www.bodynamic.ca

Bodynamic Holland*
Van Nijenrodeweg 789
1082 JJ Amsterdam
Netherlands
Tel: +31 (0)20 6611841
email: bodynamic@tiscalimail.n

Chiron

Chiron Centre*
26 Eaton Rise
London W5 2ER
UK
Tel: +44 (0)20 8997 5219
email: chiron@chiron.org

Core energetics

Institute of Core Energetics*
12th Floor
115 E 23rd Street

New York
NY 10010
USA
Tel: +1 914 228 0985
www.coreenergeticseast.org/Main.htm

Core Energetics South
8733 Lake Drive
Snellville
GA 30039
USA
Tel: +1 770 388 0086
Fax: +1 770 388 0806
email: ChubbuckPL@aol.com

Embodied-Relational Therapy

ERThWorks*
86 Burley Wood Crescent
Leeds
W Yorkshire
LS4 2QL
UK
Tel: +44 (0)845 345 8597
email: nick@erthworks.co.uk
www.erthworks.co.uk

Orgonomy

American College of Orgonomy*
PO Box 490
Princeton
NJ 08542
USA
Tel: +1 732 821 1144
Fax: +1 732 821 0174
email: aco@orgonomy.org
www.orgonomy.org/

Institute For Orgonomic Science*
205 Knapp Road
Lansdale
PA 19446
USA
Tel: +1 215 368 2678
email: annals@orgonomicscience.org

Northern California Institute for Orgonomic Therapy*
315 Eldridge Avenue
Mill Valley
CA 94941
USA
Tel: +1 415 388 0622
email: pfrisch@pacbell.net

Postural Integration/Energetic Integration

Center for Release and Integration
450 Hillside Avenue
Mill Valley
CA 94941
USA
Tel: +1 415 383 4017

Associazione di Integrazione Posturale Transpersonale
Dr Massimo Soldati
Via Scarlatti 20
20124 Milano
Italy
Tel: +39 02 2952 7815
email: maxsol@tin.it
www.web.tiscali.it/aipt_/index.htm

Institute for Bodymind Integration and Wholistic Bodywork (Belgium)
www.bodymindintegration.com/

Radix

Radix Institute*
3212 Monte Vista
NE Albuquerque
NM 87106-2120
USA
Tel: +1 888 777 2349
email: information@radix.org
www.radix.org/

Quebec Radix training*
Richard L. Cote
Université Laval
Saint Foy
PQ G1K 7P4
Canada
Tel: +418 656 2131 #2229

Somatic Emotional Therapy

Center for EnergeticStudies
2045 Francisco Street
Berkeley
CA 94709
USA
Tel: +1 510 845 8373
Fax: +1 510 841 3884
email: center@centerpress.com
www.centerpress.com

Formative Psychology
(Denmark, Germany, Greece, Netherlands, Switzerland, UK)
email: form.psy@panet.nl
www.home.wxs.nl/~form.psy/

Primal therapies

General resources

Primal Psychotherapy Page
www.webpages.charter.net/jspeyrer/

South African Primal Therapy Support Page
www.home.mweb.co.za/to/torngren/

Holotropic breathwork

Association for Holotropic Breathwork International*
PO Box 7169
Santa Cruz
CA 95061
USA
Tel: +1 650 325 4254
email: office@breathwork.com

Grof Transpersonal Training*
38 Miller Avenue
PMB 516
Mill Valley
CA 94941
USA
Tel: +1 415 383 8779
email: gtt@dnai.com
www.holotropic.com/

Primal Integration

Association for Pre- & Perinatal Psychology and Health
340 Colony Road
Geyserville
CA 95441
USA
email: apppah@aol.com
www.birthpsychology.com/

Emerson Training Seminars*
4940 Bodega Avenue
Petaluma
CA 94952
USA
Tel: +1 707 763 7024
Fax: +1 707 778 7074
www.emersonbirthrx.com/

International Society of Prenatal and Perinatal Psychology and Medicine (ISPPM)
A. & J. Bischoff
Friedhofweg 8
D-69118 Heidelberg
Germany
Tel: +49 6221 892729
Fax: +49 6221 892730
email: secretary@isppm.de
www.isppm.de/index_e.html

'Primal Scream'

The Primal Foundation (*Janov*)
1205 Abbot Kinney Boulevard
Venice
CA 90291
USA
Tel: +1 310 392 2003
Fax: +1 310 392 8554
email: primal@primaltherapy.com
www.primaltherapy.com/

International Primal Association *(not Janov)*
18 Cedar Hill Road
Ashland
MA 01721
USA
Tel: +1 877 774 6257

email: info@primals.org
www.primals.org/

London Association of Primal Therapists*
West Hill House
6 Swains Lane
London N6 6QS
UK
Tel: +44 (0)20 7267 9616
Fax: +44 (0)20 7482 0858
www.lapp.org/

Rebirthing

The Logic of Magical Thought and The Dance of the Breath (complete internet book
on Rebirthing)
www.rebirthla.com/logicintro.html

Rebirth International Online
www.rebirthingonline.com/htms/rebirth2.html

British Rebirth Society (Society for Transformational Breathwork)
General Secretary: Clare Gabriel
Tel: +44 (0)20 7722 8650
email: ClareGabriel@globalpeaceuk.com
www.users.zetnet.co.uk/rmoore/brs.html

Rebirthing New Zealand
PO Box 11-491
Wellington
New Zealand
Tel: +64 4 499 7888
Fax: +64 4 499 7884
email: info@rebirthing.co.nz

Trauma therapies

Sensorimotor therapy

Hakomi Somatics Institute*
PO Box 19438
Boulder
CO 80308
USA
Tel: +1 303 447 3290
Fax: +1 303 402 0862
email: robin@hakomisomatics.com

Somatic Experiencing

Foundation for Human Enrichment*
PO Box 1872
Lyons
CO 80540
USA
Tel: +1 303 823 9524
Fax: +1 303 823 9520
email: ergos1@earthlink.net
www.traumahealing.com/

Somatic Trauma Therapy

Center for Post-Trauma Therapy and Trauma Education*
PO Box 241783
Los Angeles
CA 90024
USA
Tel: +1 310 281 9646
Fax: +1 310 281 9729
email: babette@nwc.net
www.netppl.fi/~crisis/babrot2.htm
www.nwc.net/personal/babette/somatic.htm

Process approaches

Focusing

Focusing Institute*
34 East Lane
Spring Valley
NY 10977
USA
Tel: +1 845 362 5222
email: info@focusing.org
www.focusing.org/

Gestalt

Gestalt Therapy Page
www.gestalt.org/

International Gestalt Therapy Association
PO 1045
Highland
Y 12528-0990
USA
Tel: +1 209 671 3843
email: igta@gestalt.org

Gestalt Australia and New Zealand
www.ganz.org.au/index.html

Metanoia Trust*
13 North Common Road
Ealing
London W5 2QB
UK
Tel: +44 (0)20 8579 2505
Fax: +44 (0)20 8566 4349
www.metanoia.ac.uk

Hakomi

Hakomi Institute*
PO Box 1873
Boulder
CO 80306
USA
Tel: +1 888 421 6699
email: HakomiHQ@aol.com
www.hakomiinstitute.com/

Hakomi Institute of Europe*
Bergheimerstr 69a
69115 Heidelberg
Germany
Tel: +49 (0)6221 16 65 60
Fax: +49 (0)6221 16 66 09
email: hakomiEur@aol.com
www.hakomi.de/

Hakomi Educational Network*
PO Box 961
Ashland
OR 97520
USA
email: ron@ronkurtz.com
www.ronkurtz.com/hen.html

Process Oriented Psychology

Research Society for Process Oriented Psychology in the UK*
Tel: +44 (0)8704 295256
email: contact@rspopuk.com
www.rspopuk.com/

Process Work Center of Portland*
2049 NW Hoyt Street
Portland
OR 97209
USA
Tel: +1 503 223 8188
Fax: +1 503 227 7003
email: pwcp@igc.org
www.processwork.org/

Process Oriented Psychology Australia
Silvia Camastral
PO Box 145
Sherwood
Queensland 4075
Australia
Tel: +61 73379 4359
email: silvia@processworkaustralia.org.au
www.processworkaustralia.org.au/index.htm

Expressive therapies

Continuum

Continuum Movement*
1629 18th Street 7
Santa Monica
CA 90404
USA
Tel: +1 310 453 4402
Fax: +1 310 453 8775
email: office@continuummovement.com
www.continuummovement.com

Dance Movement Therapy

Professional Association for Dance Movement Therapy in the UK
ADMT UK
c/o Quaker Meeting House
Wedmore Vale
Bristol BS3 5HX
UK
email: query@dmtuk.demon.co.uk
www.admt.org.uk/

Pesso Boyden Psychomotor

Psychomotor Institute*
Strolling Woods on Webster Lake
Lake Shore Drive
Franklin
NH 03235
USA
Tel: +1 800 540 5548 / 603 934 5548/9809 / 603 934 0077
email: PBSP1@aol.com
www.pbsp.com/uno.htm

Voice and Voice Movement Therapy

London Voice Centre
PO Box 4218
London SE22 0JE
UK
Tel: +44 (0)20 8693 9502
email: info@voicework.com
www.voicework.com

Gale Centre
Whitakers Way
Loughton
Essex IG10 1SQ
UK
Tel: +44 (0)20 8508 9346
Fax: +44 (0)20 8502 1132
email: derek@galecent.demon.co.uk

Integrative psychotherapies

Lomi

Lomi Counseling Clinic
Waterfall Towers
Suite C-218
2455 Bennett Valley Road
Santa Rosa
CA 95404
USA
Tel: +1 707 579 0465
email: info@lomi.org
www.lomi.org/

Integrative Body Psychotherapy

Rosenberg-Kitaen Central Institute*
1551 Ocean Avenue, #230
Santa Monica
CA 90401
USA
Tel: +1 310 395-2117 or 800 IBP-2808
Fax: +1 310 395-1313
email: info@ibponline.com
www.ibponline.com/

Some other body psychotherapy centres and organizations

Centre and Institute for Psychotherapy and Emotional Bodywork*
145 Spadina Road
Toronto
Ontario M5R 2T1
Canada
Tel: +1 416 928 9570
Fax: +1 416 921 7464
email: centre@spiritcentral.com
www.spiritcentral.com/centre/

Australian College of Contemporary Somatic Therapy*
PO Box 1240
Healesville
Victoria 3777
Australia
Tel: +61 39853 2227
Fax: +61 39853 5929
email: ACCSP@somaticpsychotherapy.com.au
www.somaticpsychotherapy.com.au/

Open Centre
188 Old Street
London EC1V 9FR
Tel: +44 (0)20 8549 9583

Thinking Through The Body
Courses and seminars on neuroscience, psychoanalysis and body psychotherapy
email: info@thinkbody.co.uk
www.thinkbody.co.uk

Cambridge Centre for Body Psychotherapy*
8 Wetenhall Road
Cambridge
CB1 3AG
UK
Tel: +44 (0)1223 214658
email: gillwestland@cbpc.org.uk
www.cbpc.org.uk

London Centre for Body Psychotherapy
19 Sudbury Court Drive
Harrow
Middlesex HA1 3SZ
UK
Tel: +44 (0)20 8904 6488

Bibliography

Abrams, D. (1996) *The Spell of the Sensuous: Perception and Language in a More-Than-Human World*. New York: Pantheon.

Bainbridge Cohen, B. (1997) Body–mind centering, in D.H. Johnson (ed.) *Groundworks: Narratives of Embodiment*. Berkeley: North Atlantic Books.

Balint, M. (1968) *The Basic Fault*. London: Tavistock.

Baker, E.F. (1980) *Man in the Trap: The Causes of Blocked Sexual Energy*. New York: Collier.

Barkan, L. (1975) *Nature's Work of Art: The Human Body as Image of the World*. New Haven: Yale University Press.

Bartky, S. (1988) Foucault, femininity and the modernization of patriarchal power, in L. Quinby and I. Diamond (eds) *Feminism and Foucault: Paths of Resistance*. Boston: Northeastern University Press.

Bateson, G. (1973) *Steps to an Ecology of Mind*. St Albans: Paladin.

Bateson, G. (1980) *Mind and Nature: A Necessary Unity*. London: Fontana.

Bayer, B.M. and Malone, K.R. (1998) Feminism, psychology and matters of the body, in H.J. Stam (ed.) *The Body and Psychology*. London: Sage.

Bean, O. (1971) *Me and the Orgone: One Man's Sexual Revolution*. New York: St Martin's Press.

Behnke, E.A. (1995) Matching, in D.H. Johnson (ed.) *Groundworks: Narratives of Embodiment*. Berkeley: North Atlantic Books.

Behnke, E.A. (1997) Ghost gestures: phenomenological investigations of bodily micromovements and their intercorporeal implications, *Human Studies*, 20: 181–201.

Bentzen, M. and Bernhardt, P. (1992) *Working with Psychomotor Development*. Albany: Bodynamic Institute.

Berkowitz, L. (1999) Anger, in T. Dalgleish and M. Power (eds) *Handbook of Cognition and Emotion*. Chichester: Wiley.

Berman, M. (1990) *Coming to Our Senses: Body and Spirit in the Hidden History of the West*. London: Unwin.

Bernstein, P. (ed.) (1979) *Eight Theoretical Approaches in Dance-Movement Therapy*. Dubuque: Kendall Hunt.

Boadella, D. (ed.) (1976) *In The Wake of Reich*. London: Coventure.

Boadella, D. (1987) *Lifestreams: An Introduction to Biosynthesis*. London: Routledge & Kegan Paul.

Boadella, D. (1988) Biosynthesis, in J. Rowan and W. Dryden (eds) *Innovative Therapy in Britain*. Milton Keynes: Open University Press.

Boadella, D. (1997a) Embodiment in the therapeutic relationship, *International Journal of Psychotherapy*, 2(1): 31–44.

Boadella, D. (1997b) Awakening sensibility, recovering motility: psycho-physical synthesis at the foundations of body psychotherapy, the 100-year legacy of Pierre Janet (1859–1947), *International Journal of Psychotherapy*, 2(1): 45–56.

Bordo, S. (1993) *Unbearable Weight: Feminism, Western Culture, and the Body*. London: University of California Press.

Bourdieu, P. and Wacquant, L.J.D. (1992) *An Introduction to Reflexive Sociology*. Chicago: University of Chicago Press.

Boyesen, E. (1980) The essence of energy distribution, in G. Boyesen (ed.) *The Collected Papers of Biodynamic Psychology*. London: Biodynamic Psychology Publications.

Boyesen, G. (ed.) (1980) *The Collected Papers of Biodynamic Psychology*. London: Biodynamic Psychology Publications.

Bracken, P.J. and Petty, C. (eds) (1998) *Rethinking the Trauma of War*. London: Free Association Books.

Brittan, A. and Maynard, M. (1984) *Sexism, Racism and Oppression*. New York: Blackwell.

Brothers, L. (1997) *Friday's Footprint*. Oxford: Oxford University Press.

Brown, M. (n.d.) *The Healing Touch: An Introduction to Organismic Psychotherapy*. Self-published.

Brown, N.O. (1968) *Life Against Death: The Psychoanalytic Meaning of History*. London: Sphere.

Burkitt, I. (1999) *Bodies of Thought: Embodiment, Identity and Modernity*. London: Sage.

Cacioppo, J.T., Berntson, G.G. and Crites, S.L. Jr. (1996) Social neuroscience: principles of psychophysiological arousal and response, in E.T. Higgins and A.W. Kruglanski (eds) *Social Psychology: Handbook of Basic Principles*. New York: Guilford Press.

Cahill, L. (1997) Neurobiology of emotionally influenced memory, *Annals of the New York Academy of Sciences*, 821: 238–46.

Cameron, R. (2002) Subtle bodywork, in T. Staunton (ed.) *Body Psychotherapy*. London: Brunner-Routledge.

Carroll, R. (2001) On the border between chaos and order: the relationship between neuroscience and psychotherapy. Paper presented to the UKCP Conference 'Revolutionary Connections', London, 9 September.

Carroll, R. (2002a) Biodynamic massage in psychotherapy: re-integrating, re-owning and re-associating through the body, in T. Staunton (ed.) *Body Psychotherapy*. London: Brunner-Routledge.

Carroll, R. (2002b) Embodiment and Emotion. Seminar given to Conference on 16 April at the Tavistock Centre, London.

Casement, P. (1985) *On Learning from the Patient*. London: Routledge.

Cataldi, S.L. (1993) *Emotion, Depth and Flesh: A Study of Sensitive Space. Reflections on Merleau-Ponty's Philosophy of Embodiment*. Albany: State University of New York Press.

Chace, M. (1975) *Marion Chace: Her Papers*. Ed. H. Chaiklin. Columbia: American Dance Therapy Association.

Chaiklin, S. (1975) Dance therapy, in S. Arieti (ed.) *American Handbook of Psychiatry*, Vol. 5, 2nd edn. New York: Basic Books.

Chodorow, J. (1991) *Dance Therapy and Depth Psychology: The Moving Imagination*. London: Routledge.

Christianson, S.-A. and Engelberg, E. (1999) Organization of emotional memories, in T. Dalgleish and M. Power (eds) *Handbook of Cognition and Emotion*. Chichester: Wiley.

Cixous, H. (1994) Sonia Rykiel in translation, in S. Benstock and S. Ferriss (eds) *On Fashion*. New Brunswick, NJ: Rutgers University Press.

Cohen, D. (1995) *An Introduction to Craniosacral Therapy: Anatomy, Function, and Treatment*. Berkeley: North Atlantic Books.

Conger, J.P. (1994) *The Body in Recovery: Somatic Psychotherapy and the Self*. Berkeley: Frog.

Conrad Da'oud, E. (1995) Life on land, in D.H. Johnson (ed.) *Bone, Breath and Gesture: Practices of Embodiment*. Berkeley: North Atlantic Books.

Conrad Da'oud, E. (1997) Continuum, in D.H. Johnson (ed.) *Groundworks: Narratives of Embodiment*. Berkeley: North Atlantic Books.

Csordas, T.J. (ed.) (1994) *Embodiment and Experience: The Existential Ground of Culture and Self*. Cambridge: Cambridge University Press.

Dalgleish, T. (1999) Sadness and its disorders, in T. Dalgleish and M. Power (eds) *Handbook of Cognition and Emotion*. Chichester: Wiley.

Dalgleish, T. and Power, M. (eds) (1999) *Handbook of Cognition and Emotion*. Chichester: Wiley.

Damasio, A. (1994) *Descartes' Error: Emotion, Reason and the Human Brain*. London: PaperMac.

Damasio, A. (2000) *The Feeling of What Happens: Body, Emotion and the Making of Consciousness*. London: Heinemann.

Davidson, R.J. (1999) Neuropsychological perspectives on affective styles and their cognitive consequences, in T. Dalgleish and M. Power (eds) *Handbook of Cognition and Emotion*. Chichester: Wiley.

Davies, E. (2001) *Beyond Dance: Laban's Legacy of Movement Analysis*. Santa Ana, California: Seven Locks Press.

Davis, K. (ed.) (1997) *Embodied Practices: Feminist Perspectives on the Body*. London: Sage.

Davis, L. (1999a) Introduction and overview of the basic concepts in Radix, in L. Glenn and R. Muller-Schwefe (eds) *The Radix Reader*. Arkansas: Heron Press.

Davis, L. (1999b) Integration, in L. Glenn and R. Muller-Schwefe (eds) *The Radix Reader*. Arkansas: Heron Press.

DeMeo, J. (1998) *Saharasia: The 4000 BCE Origins of Child Abuse, Sex-Repression, Warfare and Social Violence in the Deserts of the Old World*. Ashland: Natural Energy Works.

Dychtwald, K. (1978) *Body–Mind*. New York: Jove.

Eiden, B. (2002) Application of post-Reichian body psychotherapy: a Chiron perspective, in T. Staunton (ed.) *Body Psychotherapy*. London: Brunner-Routledge.

Eigen, M. (1993) *The Electrified Tightrope*. Northvale: Jason Aronson.

Eisler, R. (1996) *Sacred Pleasure: Sex, Myth, and the Politics of the Body*. Shaftesbury: Element.

Ekman, P. (ed.) (1973) *Darwin and Facial Expression: A Century of Research in Review*. New York: Academic Press.

Ekman, P. (1999) Facial expressions, in T. Dalgleish and M. Power (eds) *Handbook of Cognition and Emotion*. Chichester: Wiley.

Engel, G. (1977) The need for a new biomedical model: a challenge for biomedicine, *Science*, 196: 164–71.

Falzeder, E. and Brabant, E. (eds) (2000) *The Correspondence of Sigmund Freud and Sandor Ferenczi*, Vol. 3: 1920–1933. Cambridge: Belknap/Harvard University Press.

Featherstone, M. (1991) The body in consumer culture, in M. Featherstone, M. Hepworth and B.S. Turner (eds) *The Body: Social Process and Cultural Theory*. London: Sage.

Featherstone, M., Hepworth, M. and Turner, B.S. (eds) (1991) *The Body: Social Process and Cultural Theory*. London: Sage.

Ferenczi, S. (1988) *The Clinical Diary*. Ed. J. Dupont. London: Harvard University Press.

Ferenczi, S. ([1930] 1999) The principle of relaxation and neo-catharsis, in J. Borossa (ed.) *Selected Writings of Sandor Ferenczi*. London: Penguin.

Fodor, N. (1949) *The Search for the Beloved*. New York: University Books.

Fogel, A. (1993) *Developing through Relationships: Origins of Communication, Self, and Culture*. Hemel Hempstead: Harvester.

Foucault, M. (1977) *Discipline and Punish: The Birth of the Prison*. London: Allen Lane.

Foucault, M. (1979) *The History of Sexuality*, Vol. 1: An Introduction. London: Allen Lane.

Frank, A.W. (1991) For a sociology of the body: an analytical review, in M. Featherstone, M. Hepworth and B.S. Turner (eds) *The Body: Social Process and Cultural Theory*. London: Sage.

Frank, A.W. (1998) From dysappearance to hyperappearance: sliding Boundaries of illness and bodies, in H.J. Stam (ed.) *The Body and Psychology*. London: Routledge.

Freud, S. (1909) Some general remarks on hysterical attacks, *Penguin Freud Library*, Vol. 10. London: Penguin.

Freud, S. (1915) Observations on transference love, *Standard Edition*, Vol. 12. London: Hogarth Press.

Freud, S. (1920) Beyond the pleasure principle, *Penguin Freud Library*, Vol. 11. London: Penguin.

Freud, S. (1923) *The Ego and the Id*. Penguin Freud Library, Vol. 11. London: Penguin.

Freud, S. (1926) Inhibitions, symptoms and anxiety, *Penguin Freud Library*, Vol. 10. London: Penguin.

Freud, S. and Breuer, J. (1893–5) Studies on hysteria. *Penguin Freud Library*, Vol. 3. London: Penguin.

Freund, P. (1982) *The Civilized Body: Social Domination, Control and Health*. Philadelphia: Temple University Press.

Freund, P. and McGuire, M. (1991) *Health, Illness and the Social Body*. Englewood Cliffs: Prentice-Hall.

Game, A. (1991) *Undoing the Social: Towards a Deconstruction of Sociology*. Buckingham: Open University Press.

Gendlin, E.T. (1981) *Focusing*. New York: Bantam.

Gendlin, E.T. (1996) *Focusing-Oriented Psychotherapy*. New York: Guilford Press.

Gibson, J.J. (1979) *The Ecological Approach to Visual Perception*. Boston: Houghton Mifflin.

Gibson, J.J. (1987) *Reasons for Realism: Selected Essays of James J. Gibson*. Eds E. Reed and R. Jones. Hillsdale: Erlbaum.

Glenn, L. and Muller-Schwefe, R. (eds) (1999) *The Radix Reader*. Arkansas: Heron Press.

Grand, I.J. (1998) Psyche's body: towards a somatic psychodynamics, in D.H. Johnson and I. J. Grand (eds) *The Body in Psychotherapy: Inquiries in Somatic Psychology*. Berkeley, CA: North Atlantic Books.

Greene, A. (1984) Giving the body its due, *Quadrant*, 17(2): 9–24.

Groddeck, G. ([1917] 1977a) Psychic conditioning and the psychoanalytic treatment of organic disorders, in L. Schacht (ed.) *The Meaning of Illness: Selected Psychoanalytic Writings by Georg Groddeck*. London: Maresfield Library.

Groddeck, G. ([1931] 1977b) Massage and psychotherapy, in L. Schacht (ed.) *The Meaning of Illness: Selected Psychoanalytic Writings by Georg Groddeck*. London: Maresfield Library.

Grof, S. (1975) *Realms of the Human Unconscious*. London: Souvenir Press.

Grossinger, R. (1995) *Planet Medicine*, 2 vols. Berkeley: North Atlantic Books.

Grossinger, R. (1998) Why somatic therapies deserve as much attention as psychoanalysis, in D.H. Johnson and I.J. Grand (eds) *The Body in Psychotherapy: Inquiries in Somatic Psychology*. Berkeley, CA: North Atlantic Books.

Grosskurth, P. (1991) *The Secret Ring: Freud's Inner Circle and the Politics of Psychoanalysis*. London: Cape.

Hancock, P., Hughes, B., Jagger, E. et al. (2000) *The Body, Culture and Society*. Buckingham: Open University Press.

Hanna, T. (1997) What is somatics?, in D.H. Johnson (ed.) *Groundworks: Narratives of Embodiment*. Berkeley, CA: North Atlantic Books.

Heckler, R.S. (1984) *The Anatomy of Change: East/West Approaches to Body/Mind Therapy*. Boston: Shambhala.

Heimann, M. (1991) Neonatal imitation: a social and biological phenomenon, in T. Archer and S. Hansen (eds) *Behavioral Biology: The Neuroendocrine Axis*. Hillsdale: Lawrence Erlbaum.

Hodge, G. (2002) Oh, you great big beautiful doll, *Independent on Sunday Living Section*, 24 February: 1–2.

House, R. and Totton, N. (eds) (1997) *Implausible Professions: Arguments for Pluralism and Autonomy in Psychotherapy and Counselling*. Hay on Wye: PCCS.

Howe, M.L., Courage, M. and Peterson, C. (1996) How can I remember when 'I' wasn't there: long-term retention of traumatic experiences and emergence of the cognitive self, in K. Pezdek and W.P. Banks (eds) *The Recovered Memory/False Memory Debate*. San Diego: Academic Press.

Hughes, B. (1999) The constitution of impairment: modernity and the aesthetic of oppression, *Disability and Society*, 14(5): 597–610.

Hughes, B. (2000) Medicalized bodies, in P. Hancock, B. Hughes, E. Jagger et al. (eds) *The Body, Culture and Society*. Buckingham: Open University Press.

Hunter, M. and Struve, J. (1997) *The Ethical Use of Touch in Psychotherapy*. London: Sage.

Iberg, J.R. (1981) Focusing, in R.J. Corsini (ed.) *Handbook of Innovative Psycho-therapies*. New York: Wiley.

Jacobs, T.J. (1973) Posture, gesture, and movement in the analyst: cues to inter-pretation and countertransference, *Journal of the American Psychoanalytic Association*, 21: 77–92.

Jacoby, M. (1986) Getting in touch and touching, in N. Schwartz-Salant and M. Stein (eds) *The Body in Analysis*. Wilmette: Chiron.

Jagger, E. (2000) Consumer bodies, in P. Hancock, B. Hughes, E. Jagger et al. (eds) *The Body, Culture and Society*. Buckingham: Open University Press.

Janet, P. (1924) *Principles of Psychotherapy*. New York: Freeport.

Janov, A. (1972) *The Primal Scream*. New York: Vintage Books.

Janov, A. (1992) *The New Primal Scream: Primal Therapy Twenty Years On*. London: Cardinal.

Johnsen, L. (1976) Muscular tonus and integrated respiration, in D. Boadella (ed.) *In the Wake of Reich*. London: Coventure.

Johnson, D.H. (ed.) (1995) *Bone, Breath and Gesture: Practices of Embodiment*. Berkeley: North Atlantic Books.

Johnson, D.H. (ed.) (1997) *Groundworks: Narratives of Embodiment*. Berkeley: North Atlantic Books.

Johnson, D.H. (2000) Intricate tactile sensitivity, *Progress Brain Research*, 122: 479–90.

Johnson, D.H. (n.d.) *The Body: Experienced and Conceptualized*. Course syllabus.

Johnson, D.H. and Grand, I.J. (eds) (1998) *The Body in Psychotherapy: Inquiries in Somatic Psychology*. Berkeley: North Atlantic Books.

Johnson, M. (1987) *The Body in the Mind: The Bodily Basis of Reason, Imagination and Reason*. Chicago: University of Chicago Press.

Johnson, S.M. (1985) *Characterological Transformation*. New York: Norton.

Jones, E. (1981) Rebirthing, in R.J. Corsini (ed.) *Handbook of Innovative Psycho-therapies*. New York: Wiley.

Juhane, D. (1987) *Job's Body: A Handbook for Bodywork*. Barrytown: Station Hill Press.

Jung, C.G. (1916) The transcendent function, *Collected Works*, Vol. 8. London: Routledge & Kegan Paul.

Jung, C.G. (1947) On the nature of the psyche, *Collected Works*, Vol. 8. London: Routledge & Kegan Paul.

Keleman, S. (1975) *Your Body Speaks Its Mind*. Berkeley: Center Press.

Keleman, S. (1976) Bio-energetic concepts of grounding, in D. Boadella (ed.) *In the Wake of Reich*. London: Coventure.

Keleman, S. (1985) *Emotional Anatomy*. Berkeley: Center Press.

Keleman, S. (1987) *Embodying Experience: Forming a Personal Life*. Berkeley: Center Press.

Kelley, C.R. (1974) *Education in Feeling and Purpose*, 2nd edn. Santa Monica: Radix Institute.

Kelley, C.R. (1976) New techniques in vision improvement, in D. Boadella (ed.) *In the Wake of Reich*. London: Coventure.

Kitamura, C. and Burnham, D. (1998) The infant's response to maternal vocal affect, in C. Rovee-Collier, L.P. Lipsett and H. Hayne (eds) *Advances in Infancy Research*, Vol. 12. Stamford: Ablex.

Klein, M. ([1930] 1998) The importance of symbol-formation in the development of the ego, in M. Klein *Love, Guilt and Reparation and Other Works*. London: Vintage.

Klein, M. ([1933] 1998) The early development of conscience in the child, in M. Klein *Love, Guilt and Reparation and Other Works*. London: Vintage.

Klein, M.H., Mathieu, P.L., Gendlin, E.T. and Kiesler, D.J. (1969) *The Experiencing Scale: A Research and Training Manual*. Madison: Wisconsin Psychiatric Institute.

Kurtz, R. (1985) *Hakomi Therapy Training Manual*. Self-published.

Kurtz, R. (1990) *Body-Centered Psychotherapy: The Hakomi Method*. Mendocino: LifeRhythm.

Kurtz, R. and Prestera, H. (1976) *The Body Reveals*. New York: Harper & Row.

Labworth, Y. and Wilson, W. (2000) Biosynthesis, *The Fulcrum*, 19: 16–19.

Lacan, J. (1977) *The Four Fundamental Concepts of Psychoanalysis*. Harmondsworth: Penguin.

Laing, R.D. (1976) *The Facts of Life*. Harmondsworth: Penguin.

Laing, R.D. (1983) *The Voice of Experience*. Harmondsworth: Penguin.

Lake, F. (1980) *Constricted Confusion*. Oxford: Clinical Theology Association.

Lakoff, G. (1987) *Women, Fire and Dangerous Things*. Chicago: University of Chicago Press.

Lakoff, G. and Johnson, M. (1980) *Metaphors We Live By*. London: University of Chicago Press.

Lakoff, G. and Johnson, M. (1999) *Philosophy in the Flesh: The Embodied Mind and its Challenge to Western Thought*. New York: Basic Books.

Lamb, W. (1965) *Posture and Gesture*. London: Duckworth.

Laplanche, J. and Pontalis, J.B. (1988) *The Language of Psychoanalysis*. London: Karnac.

Lecanuet, J.-P. (1996) Prenatal auditory experience, in I. Deliege and J. Slobada (eds) *Musical Beginnings: Origins and Development of Musical Competence*. Oxford: Oxford University Press.

LeDoux, J.E., Cicchetti, P., Xagoraris, A. and Romanski, L.R. (1990) The lateral amygdaloid nucleus: sensory interface of the amygdala in fear conditioning, *Journal of Neuroscience*, 10: 1062–9.

Leenhardt, M. ([1947] 1979) *Do Kamo: Person and Myth in a Melanesian World*. Chicago: University of Chicago Press.

Levin, D.M. (1985) *The Body's Recollection of Being: Phenomenological Psychology and the Deconstruction of Nihilism*. London: Routledge & Kegan Paul.

Levine, P.A. (1997) *Waking the Tiger: Healing Trauma*. Berkeley: North Atlantic Books.

Leys, R. (2000) *Trauma: A Genealogy*. Chicago: University of Chicago Press.

Little, M. (1990) *Psychotic Anxieties and Containment: A Personal Record of an Analysis with Winnicott*. Northvale: Jason Aronson.

Limentani, A. (1989) *Between Freud and Klein*. London: Free Association Books.

Lowen, A. (1958) *The Language of the Body* (originally published as *The Physical Dynamics of Character Structure*). New York: Collier.

Lowen, A. (1976a) *Bioenergetics*. Harmondsworth: Penguin.

Lowen, A. (1976b) Bio-energetic analysis, in D. Boadella (ed.) *In the Wake of Reich*. London: Coventure.

Lowen, A. (1977) *The Way to Vibrant Health: A Manual of Bioenergetic Exercises*. New York: Harper Colophon.

Luborsky, L., McLellan, A.T., Woody, G.E., O'Brien, C.P. and Auerbach, A. (1985) Therapists' success and its determinants, *Archives of General Psychiatry*, 42: 602–11.

Lyon, M.J. and Barbalet, J.M. (1994) Society's body, in T.J. Csordas (ed.) *Embodiment and Experience: The Existential Ground of Culture and Self*. Cambridge: Cambridge University Press.

McNeely, D.A. (1987) *Touching: Body Therapy and Depth Psychology*. Toronto: Inner City Books.

Main, M. (1999) Attachment theory: eighteen points with suggestions for future studies, in J. Cassidy and P.R. Shaver (eds) *Handbook of Attachment: Theory, Research, and Clinical Applications*. New York: Guilford Press.

Mair, K. (1992) The myth of therapist expertise, in W. Dryden and C. Feltham (eds) *Psychotherapy and its Discontents*. Buckingham: Open University Press.

Mann, D. (1997) *Psychotherapy: An Erotic Relationship*. London: Routledge.

Mann, W.E. and Hoffman, E. (1990) *Wilhelm Reich: The Man Who Dreamed of Tomorrow*. Wellingborough: Crucible.

Marcuse, H. (1966) *Eros and Civilization*. Boston: Beacon Press.

Marrone, R. (1990) *Body of Knowledge: An Introduction to Body/Mind Psychology*. Albany: State University of New York Press.

Masson, J. (1985) *The Complete Letters of Sigmund Freud to Wilhelm Fliess*. London: Belknap.

Meltzoff, A.N. and Moore, M.K. (1989) Imitation in newborn infants: exploring the range of gestures imitated and the underlying mechanisms, *Developmental Psychology*, 25: 954.

Meltzoff, A.N. and Moore, M.K. (1997) Explaining facial imitation: a theoretical model, *Early Development and Parenting*, 6: 179–92.

Miller, A. (1984) *Thou Shalt Not Be Aware*. London: Pluto Press.

Mindell, A. (1985a) *Working with the Dreaming Body*. London: Penguin Arkana.

Mindell, A. (1985b) *River's Way: The Process Science of the Dreambody*. London: Penguin Arkana.

Mindell, A. (1988) *Dreambody*. London: Penguin Arkana.

Mindell, A. (1990) *Working On Yourself Alone: Inner Dreambody Work*. London: Penguin Arkana.

Mindell, A. (1993) *The Shaman's Body: A New Shamanism for Transforming Health, Relationships, and the Community*. San Francisco, CA: Harper Collins.

Mindell, A. (1995) *Metaskills*. Scottsdale: New Falcon.

Mindell, A. and Mindell, A. (1992) *Riding the Horse Backward: Process Work in Theory and Practice*. London: Penguin Arkana.

Montagu, A. (1971) *Touching: The Human Significance of the Skin*. New York: Harper & Row.

Mott, F. (1959) *The Nature of the Self*. London: Allen Wingate.

Mowbray, R. (1995) *The Case Against Psychotherapy Registration: A Conservation Issue for the Human Potential Movement*. London: Trans Marginal Press.

Neafsey, E.J. (1990) Prefrontal cortical control of the autonomic nervous system: anatomical and physiological observations, *Progress in Brain Research*, 85: 147–66.

Newham, P. (1999) *Using Voice and Movement in Therapy: The Practical Application of Voice Movement Therapy*. London: Jessica Kingsley.

Nietzsche, F. (1978) *Thus Spake Zarathustra*. Harmondsworth: Penguin.

Ofshe, R. and Watters, E. (1994) *Making Monsters: False Memories, Psychotherapy, and Sexual Hysteria*. New York: Scribners.

Ogden, P. and Minton, K. (2000) Sensorimotor psychotherapy: one method for processing traumatic memory, *Traumatology: An Online Journal*, 6(3) Article 3: http://www.fsu.edu/~trauma/v6i3/v6i303.html

Orr, L. and Ray, S. (1983) *Rebirthing in the New Age*. Berkeley: Celestial Arts.

Oschman, J.L. (2000) *Energy Medicine: The Scientific Basis*. Edinburgh: Churchill Livingstone.

Ots, T. (1994) The silenced body – the expressive Leib: on the dialectic of mind and life in Chinese cathartic healing, in T.J. Csordas (ed.) *Embodiment and Experience: The Existential Ground of Culture and Self*. Cambridge: Cambridge University Press.

Painter, J.W. (1984) *Deep Bodywork and Personal Development: Harmonizing Our Bodies, Emotions and Thoughts*. Mill Valley: Center for Release and Integration.

Panksepp, J. (1998) *Affective Neuroscience: The Foundations of Human and Animal Emotions*. Oxford: Oxford University Press.

Partington, A. (ed.) (1996) *Oxford Dictionary of Quotations*, 4th edn. Oxford: Oxford University Press.

Peerbolte, M.L. (1975) *Psychic Energy*. Wassenaar: Servire.

Perls, F. (1955) Gestalt therapy and human potentialities, in J.O. Stevens (ed.) *Gestalt Is*. New York: Bantam.

Perls, F. ([1947] 1969) *Ego, Hunger and Aggression*. New York: Vintage Books.

Perls, F., Hefferline, R.F. and Goodman, P. ([1951] 1973) *Gestalt Therapy: Excitement and Growth in the Human Personality*. Harmondsworth: Penguin.

Perry, B.D. (1997) Memories of fear: how the brain stores and retrieves physiologic states, feelings, behaviors and thoughts from traumatic events, in J. Goodwin and R. Attias (eds) *Images of the Body in Trauma*. New York: Basic Books.

Perry, B.D. and Marcellus, J. (1997) *The Impact of Abuse and Neglect on the Developing Brain*. Houston: CIVITAS.

Perry, B.D. and Pollard, R. (1998) Homeostasis, stress, trauma and adaptation: a neurodevelopmental view of childhood trauma, *Child and Adolescent Psychiatric Clinics of North America*, 7(1): 33–49.

Perry, B.D., Pollard, R., Blakley, T.L., Baker, W.L. and Vigilante, D. (1995) Childhood trauma, the neurobiology of adaptation, and 'use-dependent' development of the brain: how 'states' become 'traits', *Infant Mental Health Journal*, 16(4): 271–91.

Pert, C. (1986) The wisdom of the receptors: neuropeptides, the emotions and the bodymind, *Advances: The Journal of Body–Mind Health*, 3(3): 8–16.

Pesso, A. (1973) *Experience in Action*. New York: New York University Press.

Phillips, A. (1994) *On Flirtation*. London: Faber & Faber.

Pierrakos, J. (1987) *Core Energetics: Developing the Capacity to Love and Heal*. Mendocino: LifeRhythm.

Pitzal, W. (1999) The Radix approach: a brief description, in L. Glenn and R. Muller-Schwefe (eds) *The Radix Reader*. Arkansas: Heron Press.

Polster, E. and Polster, M. (1974) *Gestalt Therapy: Integrated Contours of Theory and Practice*. New York: Vintage.

Porges, S.W. (1995) Orienting in a defensive world: mammalian modifications of our evolutionary heritage. A polyvagal theory, *Psychophysiology*, 32: 301–18.

Porges, S.W. (1997) Emotion: an evolutionary by-product of the neural regulation of the autonomic nervous system, *Annals of the New York Academy of Sciences*, 807: 62–77.

Porges, S.W. and Bazhenova, O.V. (n.d.) Evolution and the autonomic nervous system: a neurobiological model of socio-emotional and communication disorders. http://www.icdl.com/porges.html

Prescott, J. (1971) Early somatosensory deprivation as an ontogenetic process in the abnormal development of the brain and behavior, in E.I. Goldsmith and J. Moor-Janowski (eds) *Medical Primatology*. New York: Karger.

Prescott, J. (1975) Body pleasure and the origins of violence, *Bulletin of Atomic Scientists*, November: 10–20.

Proust, M. (2000) *Time Regained*, tr. C.K. Scott Montoneff and T. Kilmartin, revised D.J. Enright. London: Vintage.

Prout, A. (ed.) (2000) *The Body, Childhood and Society*. London: Macmillan.

Raknes, O. (1971) *Wilhelm Reich and Orgonomy: The Controversial Theory of Life Energy*. Baltimore: Penguin.

Ramsden, P. (1992) The action profile system of movement assessment for self development, in H. Payne (ed.) *Dance Movement Therapy: Theory and Practice*. London: Routledge.

Rank, O. ([1929] 1993) *The Trauma of Birth*. New York: Dover.

Reich, W. (1960) *Selected Writings*. New York: Farrar, Straus Giroux.

Reich, W. ([1948] 1967) *Listen, Little Man!* New York: Farrar, Straus Giroux.

Reich, W. ([1945] 1972) *Character Analysis*. New York: Touchstone.

Reich, W. ([1950] 1972) *Ether, God and Devil*. New York: Farrar, Straus Giroux.

Reich, W. ([1942] 1983) *The Function of the Orgasm*. London: Souvenir.

Romanes, G.J. (1978) *Cunningham's Textbook of Anatomy*. Oxford: Oxford University Press.

Rosenberg, J.L. and Rand, M.L. (1985) *Body, Self, and Soul: Sustaining Integration*. Atlanta: Humanics.

Rosenberg, V. (1995) On touching a patient, *British Journal of Psychotherapy*, 12(1): 29–36.

Roth, A. and Fonagy, P. (1996) *What Works for Whom? A Critical Review of Psychotherapy Research*. London: Guilford Press.

Rothschild, B. (2000) *The Body Remembers: The Psychophysiology of Trauma and Trauma Treatment*. New York: Norton.

Rowan, J. (1988) Primal integration therapy, in J. Rowan and W. Dryden (eds) *Innovative Therapy in Britain*. Milton Keynes: Open University Press.

Rowan, J. and Dryden, W. (1988) *Innovative Therapy in Britain*. Milton Keynes: Open University Press.

Rozin, P., Haidt, J. and McCauley, C.R. (1999) Disgust, in T. Dalgleish and M. Power (eds) *Handbook of Cognition and Emotion*. Chichester: Wiley.

Russell, R. (2000) Ethical bodies, in P. Hancock, B. Hughes, E. Jagger et al. *The Body, Culture and Society*. Buckingham: Open University Press.

Sampson, E.E. (1998) Establishing embodiment in psychology, in H.J. Stam (ed.) *The Body and Psychology*. London: Sage.

Samuels, A. (1989) *The Plural Psyche: Personality, Morality and the Father*. London: Routledge.

Schoop, T. (1974) *Won't You Join the Dance?* Palo Alto: National Press Books.

Schore, A.N. (1994) *Affect Regulation and the Origin of the Self: The Neurobiology of Emotional Development*. Mahwah: Erlbaum.

Schore, A.N. (2001a) Contributions from the decade of the brain to infant mental health: an overview, *Infant Mental Health Journal*, 22(1–2): 1–6.

Schore, A.N. (2001b) Effects of a secure attachment relationship on right brain development, affect regulation, and infant mental health, *Infant Mental Health Journal*, 22(1–2): 7–66.

Schore, A.N. (2001c) The effects of early relational trauma on right brain development, affect regulation, and infant mental health, *Infant Mental Health Journal*, 22(1–2): 201–69.

Schwartz-Salant, N. (1982) *Narcissism and Character-Transformation: The Psychology of Narcissistic Character Disorders*. Toronto: Inner City Books.

Schwartz-Salant, N. and Stein, M. (eds) (1986) *The Body in Analysis*. Wilmette: Chiron.

Seeman, J. (1996) Level of experiencing and psychotherapy outcome, *The Folio: A Journal for Focusing and Experiential Therapy*, 15: 15–18.

Seligman, M.E.P. (1995) The effectiveness of psychotherapy: the consumer reports study, *American Psychologist*, 50(12): 965–74.

Sharaf, M. (1984) *Fury on Earth: A Biography of Wilhelm Reich*. London: Hutchinson.

Sheets-Johnstone, M. (1990) *The Roots of Thinking*. Philadelphia: Temple University Press.

Shilling, C. (1993) *The Body and Social Theory*. London: Sage.

Siegel, E.V. (1984) *Dance-Movement Therapy: Mirror of Our Selves; The Psychoanalytic Approach*. New York: Human Sciences Press.

Smith, E.W.L. (1985) *The Body in Psychotherapy*. Jefferson: McFarland.

Solms, M. and Turnbull, O. (2002) *The Brain and the Inner World: An Introduction to the Neuroscience of Subjective Experience*. London: Karnac.

Southgate, J. (1980) Basic dimensions of character analysis, *Energy and Character*, 11(1): 48–67.

Southwell, C. (1988) The Gerda Boyesen method: biodynamic therapy, in J. Rowan and W. Dryden (eds) *Innovative Therapy in Britain*. Milton Keynes: Open University Press.

Spiegelman, J.M. (1992) *Reich, Jung, Regardie and Me: The Unhealed Healer*. Scottsdale: New Falcon.

Spiegelman, J.M. (1996) *Psychotherapy as Mutual Process*. Scottsdale: New Falcon.

Stam, H.J. (ed.) (1998) *The Body and Psychology*. London: Sage.

Stanton-Jones, K. (1992) *An Introduction to Dance Movement Therapy in Psychiatry*. London: Routledge.

Staunton, T. (2002) Sexuality and body psychotherapy, in T. Staunton (ed.) *Body Psychotherapy*. London: Brunner-Routledge.

Stern, D. (1985) *The Interpersonal World of the Infant*. New York: Basic Books.

Stevens, B. (1977) Body work, in J.O. Stevens (ed.) *Gestalt Is*. New York: Bantam.

Taylor, G.J. (1992) Psychosomatics and self-regulation, in J.W. Barron, M.N. Eagle and D.L. Wolitzky (eds) *Interface of Psychoanalysis and Psychology*. Washington, DC: American Psychological Association.

Taylor, K. (1994) *The Breathwork Experience: Exploration and Healing in Nonordinary States of Consciousness*. Santa Cruz: Hanford Mead.

Totton, N. (1998) *The Water in the Glass: Body and Mind in Psychoanalysis*. London: Rebus.

Totton, N. (1999) The baby and the bathwater: 'professionalisation' in psychotherapy and counselling, *British Journal of Guidance and Counselling*, 27(3): 313–24.

Totton, N. (2000) *Psychotherapy and Politics*. London: Sage.

Totton, N. (2002a) Foreign bodies: recovering the history of body psychotherapy, in T. Staunton (ed.) *Body Psychotherapy*. London: Brunner-Routledge.

Totton, N. (2002b) The future for body psychotherapy, in T. Staunton (ed.) *Body Psychotherapy*. London: Brunner-Routledge.

Totton, N. and Edmondson, E. (1988) *Reichian Growth Work: Melting the Blocks to Life and Love*. Bridport: Prism Press (available on the internet via http://www.erthworks.co.uk).

Totton, N. and Jacobs, M. (2001) *Character and Personality Types*. Buckingham: Open University Press.

Trevarthen, C. (1993) The self born in intersubjectivity: the psychology of an infant communicating, in U. Neisser (ed.) *The Perceived Self: Ecological and Interpersonal Sources of Self-knowledge*. New York: Cambridge University Press.

Trevarthen, C. (2001) Intrinsic motives for companionship in understanding: their origin, development, and significance for infant mental health, *Infant Mental Health Journal*, 22: 1–2.

Trevarthen, C. and Aitken, K.J. (2001) Infant intersubjectivity: research, theory and clinical applications, *Journal of Child Psychology and Psychiatry*, 42(1): 3–48.

Turner, B.S. (1984) *The Body and Society: Explorations in Social Theory*. Oxford: Blackwell.

Turner, B.S. (1991) Recent developments in the theory of the body, in M. Featherstone, M. Hepworth and B.S. Turner (eds) *The Body: Social Process and Cultural Theory*. London: Sage.

Turner, B.S. (1992) *Regulatory Bodies: Essays in Medical Sociology*. London: Routledge.

Turner, E.-J. (1998) The Hakomi method of body-centred psychotherapy: its contribution to the evolution of the character map, *Self and Society*, 26(4): 11–16.

Turner, T. (1994) Bodies and anti-bodies, in T.J. Csordas (ed.) *Embodiment and Experience: The Existential Ground of Culture and Self*. Cambridge: Cambridge University Press.

Turp, M. (2001) *Psychosomatic Health: the Body and the Word*. London: Palgrave.

Ukleja, K. (1998) Inertia, entropy and the eye of the needle, *Rhythm and News: Craniosacral Therapy Association Journal*, 13: 4–5.

Van der Kolk, B. (1994) The body keeps the score: memory and the evolving psychobiology of post traumatic stress, *Harvard Review of Psychiatry*, 1(5): 253–65.

VanOyen Witvliet, C. (1997) Traumatic intrusive imagery as an emotional memory phenomenon: a review of research and explanatory information processing theories, *Clinical Psychology Review*, 17: 509–36.

Varela, F., Thompson, E. and Rosch, E. (1992) *The Embodied Mind*. Cambridge: MIT Press.

Vick, P. (2002) Psycho-spiritual body psychotherapy, in T. Staunton (ed.) *Body Psychotherapy*. London: Brunner-Routledge.

West, W. (1994) Clients' experience of bodywork psychotherapy, *Counselling Psychology Quarterly*, 7(3): 287–303.

Winnicott, D.W. ([1947] 1987a) Hate in the countertransference, in D.W. Winnicott *Through Paediatrics to Psychoanalysis: Collected Papers*. London: Karnac.

Winnicott, D.W. ([1949] 1987b) Mind and its relation to the psyche-soma, in D.W. Winnicott *Through Paediatrics to Psychoanalysis: Collected Papers*. London: Karnac.

Winnicott, D.W. ([1954] 1987a) Metapsychological and clinical aspects of regression within the psychoanalytical set-up, in D.W. Winnicott *Through Paediatrics to Psychoanalysis: Collected Papers*. London: Karnac.

Young, C. and Heller, M. (2000) The scientific 'what!' of psychotherapy: psychotherapy is a craft, not a science, *International Journal of Psychotherapy*, 5(2): 113–31.

Young, R.M. (1994) *Mental Space*. London: Process Press.

Index

CHARACTER AND PERSONALITY TYPES

Nick Totton and Michael Jacobs

It is very difficult for the student or practitioner to find their way through the jungle of different personality typographies that has sprung up in the field of psychotherapy; and even harder for them to find a point of sufficient height above the forest canopy to get their bearings in order to compare one system with another. This volume offers such an observation point together with some possible mappings. It surveys how different schools of therapy approach a basic topic, the differences that exist between people – including their attitudes, feelings, concerns and talents. It examines different systematic and non-systematic approaches to identifying different types of human being, exploring whether there are systematic ways in which humans vary, how we can assess the merit of different typologies, and whether personality typing is a helpful approach to therapy.

Character and Personality Types looks in detail at the arguments for and against the use of typologies of character and personality as a clinical tool; and offers general criteria for judging the merits of particular personality systems, as well as exploring the possibility of a wider synthesis.

Contents
Orientations – Character in psychoanalysis – Reich and his heirs – Jungian typology – Humanistic and research based typologies – Transpersonal typologies – Conclusion – Further reading – References – Index.

c.128pp   0 335 20639 5 (Paperback)   0 335 20640 9 (Hardback)

AN INTRODUCTION TO COUNSELLING
Third Edition

John McLeod (editor)

Reviews of the second edition:

It is impossible to do justice to such an exhaustive, broad-based and very readable work in a short review. Professor McLeod has been meticulous, and with true scientific impartiality has looked at, studied and described the many strands and different schools of thought and methods that can lead towards successful counselling.

Therapy Weekly

This is a fascinating, informative, comprehensive and very readable book . . . McLeod has produced a text that offers a great deal no matter what your level of competence or knowledge.

Journal of Interprofessional Care

One of the book's strengths is McLeod's willingness to go beyond a history of the development of counselling or a beginner's technical manual . . . [and to] consider the political dimensions of counselling and the relevance of power to counselling relationships. A worthwhile acquisition for therapeutic community members, whatever their discipline or background.

Therapeutic Communities

This thoroughly revised and expanded version of the best-selling text *An Introduction to Counselling* provides a comprehensive introduction to the theory and practice of counselling and therapy. It is written in a clear, accessible style, covers all the core approaches to counselling, and takes a critical, questioning approach to issues of professional practice. Placing each counselling approach in its social and historical context, the book also introduces a wide range of contemporary approaches, including narrative therapy, systemic, feminist and multicultural.

This third edition includes a new chapter on the important emerging approach of philosophical counselling, and a chapter on the counselling relationship, as well as expanded coverage of attachment theory, counselling on the Internet, and solution-focused therapy. The text has been updated throughout, with additional illustrative vignettes and case studies.

Current, comprehensive and readable, *An Introduction to Counselling* is a classic introduction to its subject.

c.464pp   0 335 21189 5 (Paperback)   0 335 21190 9 (Hardback)